A Balm for Gilead

A Balm for Gilead

Meditations on Spirituality and the Healing Arts

DANIEL P. SULMASY, O.F.M., M.D.

GEORGETOWN UNIVERSITY PRESS / Washington, D.C.

As of January 1, 2007, 13-digit ISBN numbers will replace the current 10-digit system.
Paperback: 13: 978-1-58901-122-9

Georgetown University Press, Washington, D.C.

Library of Congress Cataloging-in-Publication Data

Sulmasy, Daniel P., 1956–
    A balm for Gilead : meditations on spirituality and the healing arts / by Daniel P. Sulmasy.
        p. ; cm.
    Includes bibliographical references.
    ISBN-13: 978-1-58901-122-9 (pbk. : alk. paper)
    ISBN-10: 1-58901-122-8 (pbk. : alk. paper)
    1. Medical ethics.   2. Medicine—Religious aspects.   3. Spirituality.
I. Title.
    [DNLM: 1. Physician's Role—psychology.   2. Spirituality.
3. Catholicism—psychology.   4. Patient Care—ethics.   5. Religion
and Medicine. W 62 S233b 2006]
    R725.55.S85   2006
    174.2—dc22

                                                                2006006700

This book is printed on acid-free paper meeting the requirements of the American National Standard for Permanence in Paper for Printed Library Materials.

13 12 11 10 09 08 07 06   9 8 7 6 5 4 3 2
First printing

Printed in the United States of America

For the people of All Saints Parish,
Harlem, U.S.A.

You inspire me more than you know.

Contents

Preface

> Is there no balm in Gilead? Is there no physician here?
> Why then has the health of my poor people not been restored?
>
> —JEREMIAH 8:22

W HEN I wrote *The Healer's Calling: A Spirituality for Physicians and Other Health Care Professionals* (Paulist Press) in 1997, spirituality was something almost never discussed in medical circles. Much has changed since then. Thanks in large part to a funding initiative sponsored by the Templeton Foundation, most U.S. medical schools now have established courses in spirituality and health care. Articles about the topic now appear regularly in medical journals. Conferences on spirituality and health care are held all over the country multiple times each year. Newspapers and magazines have given the topic prominent local and national coverage.

These developments have not been uncontroversial, however. A cadre of fierce critics has attacked the entire idea of introducing (or, perhaps better, reintroducing) spirituality into medicine as a violation of the profession's unwritten constitutional directive commanding the separation of church and clinic. Even religious thinkers have been divided on just how religion should be incorporated into health care, if at all. Some chaplains have feared that this movement represents a failure on the part of the "medical establishment" to appreciate pastoral care's unique expertise and contribution to health care. Empirical studies have dominated the medical literature on the role of religion and spirituality in health care, but these studies have been alternately championed and ridiculed as bad science.

Recently, I published a book that plunged into these controversies— *The Rebirth of the Clinic: An Introduction to Spirituality in Health Care* (Georgetown University Press, 2006). That book addressed broad issues,

such as the definition of spirituality, the nature of the relationship between the spiritual and the clinical, the scope (and limits) of empirical
research about spirituality in health care, and the ethics of incorporat-
ing attention to patient spirituality into clinical practice. It was addressed to a fairly wide audience. Although deeply influenced by my
own faith commitments, it was not expressly confessional. Affective or
inspirational passages were included solely with the aim of explicating
the spiritual possibilities inherent in clinical practice. In other words,
The Rebirth of the Clinic was a book *about* spirituality in health care.

By contrast, *A Balm for Gilead* is a work *of* spirituality. It is addressed
primarily to persons of faith (particularly Christians) or those who are
exploring their own faith commitments. It is a book written primarily
for health care professionals, but I hope it will also be useful to those
who are themselves sick or dying or caring for loved ones who are sick
or are dying. It is a series of meditations, not explanations. It is intended to inspire more than to instruct.

Nonetheless, the spirituality presented here is far from mindless.
The text moves back and forth between the affective, the poetic, and the
speculative. Some may find such movement jarring. They may expect
theology to be intellectually rigorous and expect spirituality to be moving and motivational. Subsequently, a spirituality that is speculative or
a theology that is inspirational may appear disjointed. I am convinced,
however, that such divisions are dangerous. Just as genuine spirituality
cannot ignore this world in favor of the world to come, so genuine
spirituality cannot ignore the rational in favor of the affective. I do not
believe God made us as creatures divided thus asunder. I do not believe
we are under any compulsion to check our brains in at a jar by the door
before entering the sanctuary; nor do I believe we should extirpate our
hearts before we enter the theology library. Many of the greatest spiritual writers—Augustine and Bonaventure come to mind—freely ad-
mixed the spiritual and the speculative. I profess to equal neither of
these spiritual giants. But I would invite the reader who is troubled by
these stylistic shifts to bear in mind that the reason this book traverses
both the speculative and the affective is that I am convinced that the
mind and the heart are united in the fully Christian person.

Some readers might have misgivings about a book like this being
written by a professor of medicine rather than by a chaplain or a pastor.
My protestations about the need to unite the affective and the rational
aside, one must admit that the worlds of spirituality and academia have

never had an easy relationship. In the Gospels, Jesus praises the God who has "hidden these things from the wise and the intelligent and [has] revealed them to infants" (Mt 11:25). St. Francis of Assisi distrusted academics, citing St. Paul's familiar admonitions that "knowledge puffs up" (1 Cor 8:1) and that "the letter kills, but the spirit gives life" (2 Cor 3:6).

One must concede that sometimes it does seem easier for persons who are neither intellectually gifted nor academically advantaged to become holy. Those who have had access to education may face spiritual stumbling blocks such as pride or similar barriers created out of their own intelligence and academic experience. Schooling is also often associated with the kind of social advantage that can make people forget their dependence on God. And so, there is substantial truth to the precaution that entering the kingdom of God may be more difficult for those who take a torturous intellectual route.

Yet a number of peculiar difficulties arise for anyone who would write a book about spirituality, whether an academician or not. To the extent that spirituality is any kind of knowing, it is the knowing of familiarity rather than the knowing of facts. It is not the knowing of propositions and formulae (knowing that) or the knowing of technique (knowing how). For those who share my faith that the transcendent is a person, spirituality is really a knowing Who.

Writing a book *of* spirituality therefore requires me to be confessional. The Who I believe I need to know is Jesus Christ. Accordingly, most of the chapters of this book are explicitly religious. They rely heavily on texts from Christian scripture and the writings of the saints. At some junctures, their purpose is to prick the consciences of those who claim to be followers of Christ and practitioners of the healing arts. At other points, they take up the call of St. Francis that a friar should become a minstrel for God, touching the hearts of the faithful and raising them to spiritual joy.

Writing a book about health care that assumes a faith perspective may be unfashionable, but it is simply not possible to "do" spirituality without assuming an explicit, personal perspective. This is not a book about dogma, but an exploration of the spiritual dimensions of health care. As such, it necessarily draws heavily on my personal experience as a Christian physician. My own spiritual life, like that of most spiritual persons, has been formed and nurtured within the context of my faith. I do not pretend to know enough about other religions or about nonreligious approaches to spirituality to theologize about them. I do know, however, that the core concepts of Catholic Christianity touch on the most central aspects of what it means to be a human being. Persons of other faiths or of no faith usually find that they can understand what I am trying to say if I seek to understand the meaning of my own faith in the context of my own medical and spiritual practices.

Spirituality is about transcendent relationship. The aim of a work of spirituality is to help the reader to know self, God, and neighbor more deeply. I offer this book as a step down the path, however crooked and human it may be, toward God's own dream of universal right relationship, in every place and for every time. That is everything that a work of spirituality in health care could ever hope to accomplish.

Since the publication of *The Healer's Calling*, I am aware of only two other books that have looked directly at the spirituality of those who provide professional care for the sick—*The Nurse's Calling: A Christian Spirituality of Caring for the Sick* by Mary Elizabeth O'Brien (Paulist Press, 2001) and, at least in part, John Shea's *Spirituality and Health Care* (Park Ridge Center for the Study of Health, Faith, and Ethics, 2000). I find this lack of attention to the spirituality of health care professionals both surprising and not surprising. It is surprising in light of the fact that spiritual issues arise in all occupations, that there is a growing movement of workplace spirituality in the United States, and that the various health professions have recently become intensely aware of the spiritual concerns of those they serve. One would have thought it obvious that authors grappling with questions of spirituality and the care of patients would have been thinking more about the spiritual needs of the health care professionals themselves. Nevertheless, this lack of attention to the spirituality of health care professionals is not so surprising if one understands health care professionals. The scientific culture of health care often denigrates subjects that are classified as "soft." This broad brush of "softness" is wiped across a canvas that includes subjects such as public health, professional-patient communication, the history of medicine, medical sociology, and medical ethics. Many of these subjects strive for legitimacy by presenting themselves in as "scientific" a light as possible, designating other, less quantitative subjects as the "truly soft" topics, thereby painting themselves within the core of medicine. Epidemiologists have been quite successful in this endeavor. By emphasizing molecular epidemiology and their mastery of statistics and pointing to other subjects as "soft," epidemiologists have earned their place at the medical table. Spirituality, of course, is the ultimate "soft" subject in health care. Because there is no subject that could be considered "softer," this trick will not work for spirituality. The buck stops here.

In addition, the health professions have long emphasized a certain mental toughness that, although quite functional and healthy in many ways, can sometimes lead to a dysfunctional and unhealthy hardness of heart—a denial of one's own feelings and aspirations as well as those of one's colleagues. Thus, to admit that one was in the throes of a personal spiritual struggle would be, in many medical circles, considered a sign of weakness. To ask how a loving God could allow patients to suffer would not be a question the attending physician would welcome on rounds. To suggest praying for a patient or a colleague might be considered a way of asking to be transferred from the University Hospital to the St. Elsewhere's residency training program.

Yet, if one of the main theses of this book is correct, this is tantamount to denying the deepest aspects of one's own humanity and the actual meaning of one's work. Given the self-doubt, crises in professional identity, and the iatrogenic burdens that medical technology brings on those who deploy it as well as those who are served by it, health care professionals are now experiencing an ever greater need for spiritual succor. This book is devoted to the diagnosis of the spiritual malaise of physicians, nurses, and other health care professionals and to the exploration of how Christian healers can be inspired by the vision of the Gospel to persevere in the care of the sick.

These themes weave their way forward in a manner that is ultimately systematic, even if it is alternately inspirational and investigational, affective and rational. I have already mentioned that the subject requires all these perspectives. Health care professionals inhabit multiple spheres of discourse, and spirituality touches them all. The urge to compartmentalize spirituality is part of the problem spirituality must address. These pieces must all fit together if one is to see the whole.

I begin the book with a reflection on the relationship between spirituality and morality in clinical practice and point out that the spiritual cannot be reduced to the moral. To illustrate this in a dramatic way, in chapter 2 I present a meditation that I call "Letter to a Young Intern," inspired by a letter of Thomas Merton. I then provide, in chapter 3, an understanding of the meaning of healing in Catholic Christianity.

Chapter 4 is about those who are physically unattractive and the responsibilities health care professionals have toward them. I then probe,
in chapter 5, the present spiritual malaise of health care professionals
and in chapters 6 and 7 consider several passages of Christian scripture
in light of the question of the relationship between sinfulness, sickness,
and suffering. Moving from the diagnostic to the therapeutic mode, in
chapter 8 I suggest how the wisdom of the Beatitudes might help clinicians and in chapter 9 how the wisdom of St. Francis and his early
followers could point the way to a twenty-first-century spirituality for
health care professionals. In chapter 10, I move from the acute care
setting to primary care and suggest a spiritual understanding of preventive medicine as stewardship of the body. Chapter 11 considers the
spirituality of death in the light of Christian hope, and chapter 12 follows as a meditation for those who mourn the loss of their loved ones.
I conclude the book with a prayer.

Writing this book has not been easy. My primary academic work is in
medical ethics, not spirituality. I continue to see patients and to teach
medical students, residents, and fellows. Given the many hats I wear, I
could not have written this book without the help of many people, and
I would like to recognize some of them.

First, I would like to thank Father Patrick Primeaux and the Theology Department of St. John's University for offering me the McKeever
Chair in Moral Theology, where I served as a visiting professor from
September 2003 through December 2004. I am very grateful to Sidney
Callahan, my predecessor in the McKeever Chair, for suggesting my
name to St. John's. I especially thank Lynn Jansen, who ably picked up
so many of my responsibilities at St. Vincent's Hospital–Manhattan
and at New York Medical College, enabling me to devote time to this
book and to other writing projects. I am also enormously grateful to
Dr. Alan Astrow, who read this entire manuscript and offered his cri-
tique. I suppose that spouses often do this for other writers. In New
York City in the twenty-first century, it takes a sincerely pious Jewish
oncologist to help a Franciscan internist and philosopher write a book
about God.

I have also greatly benefited from the comments of two reviewers for
Georgetown University Press—both the one who chose to disclose his
identity, Farr Curlin, M.D., and the one who remained anonymous.

Their insights and detailed attention to the text have helped enormously in shaping this book.

Finally, I wish to thank the people of All Saints Parish in Harlem, New York. My gratitude starts at home, with my brother friars, Charlie Gilmartin, Glenn Humphrey, Chris Keenan, Neil O'Connell, and Ben Taylor. It is a simple fact that the spiritual life is much easier when undertaken with others who are dedicated to prayer, fraternal support, and service.

Yet the secret of All Saints Parish is the congregation. The faith of the people of Harlem inspires me and evangelizes me. I am grateful that they have allowed a community of friars to live among them. Much to my surprise, since moving to this parish three years ago I have grown to love Gospel music, to understand fully how one can sing it well only if one sincerely believes it, and to appreciate how deeply Catholic the singing of African-American Gospel music can be. Each Sunday, before the dismissal rite of the mass, those who are charged with bringing communion to the sick and shut-ins of the parish are blessed by Father Neil and the congregation. During that blessing, week in and week out, we sing a version of an African-American spiritual:

There is a balm in Gilead
To make the wounded whole.
There is a balm in Gilead
To heal the sin-sick soul.

We all need to find that balm—whether we are physicians, nurses, psychologists, or patients. We need it for the sake of those we serve. We need it for ourselves.

I cannot pray like Peter. I cannot preach like Paul. But I can tell all the folks in Gilead that there is balm enough for all.

A Balm for Gilead

CHAPTER 1

The Numinous, the Medical, and the Moral

> Being Christian is not the result of an ethical choice or a lofty idea, but the encounter with an event, a person, which gives life a new horizon and a decisive direction.
>
> BENEDICT XVI, *Deus Caritas Est*

FOR the last five years one of my colleagues, Dr. Alan Astrow, and I have been running a series of conferences at St. Vincent's Hospital–Manhattan that we have called "Spirituality, Religious Wisdom, and the Care of the Patient."[1] We have brought together clinicians and religious thinkers to discuss spiritual issues that commonly arise in clinical care. In an effort to make this a fully ecumenical, interfaith enterprise, each session features two religious speakers of different religious backgrounds. The series has been enormously successful and always draws great crowds. I have been surprised, however, by one problem that we have encountered consistently: Every clinician we involve in the program seems to conflate spirituality and ethics. When we ask for suggestions about spiritual topics for the program, they always suggest ethical topics. When we ask for suggestions about potential speakers for a series about spirituality, they always suggest ethicists. And when we ask for cases for our discussions that illustrate some of the spiritual issues that arise in practice, they always hand us crisply written clinical ethics cases, ones that are "thin" enough to be suitable for presentation at medical grand rounds. More often than not, "the spiritual problem" chosen is a case of a religiously fundamentalist family from a minority racial group praying for a "miracle" and refusing to authorize the withholding or withdrawing of life-sustaining treatments when the doctors and nurses all know that the patient will not survive to hospital discharge.

A central thesis of this book is that this approach reveals a profound misunderstanding of what spirituality means. Spirituality is not ethics. Yet the intuition that spirituality and ethics are somehow related is not entirely mistaken.

In part, the conflation of the spiritual with the ethical might reveal a deep suspicion on the part of clinicians that all ethics is actually religious. For some, this suspicion raises a troubling logical concatenation—namely, "Ethics means religion, and religion means a lot of up-tight people telling me what I can't do." Because they do not wish to be told what to do, they reject both the spiritual and the ethical.

For another subset, the idea that spirituality implies ethics is a good thing. It may indicate an explicit belief that religion is the only true source of morality. Or it may reflect an inchoate understanding, not conscious or explicit, that their own personal moralities have been deeply influenced by their own individual religious upbringings, whether or not they actually practice that religion at present.

The notion that all ethics is ultimately religious is, in fact, both true and false. It is false in the sense that philosophical ethics is a discipline that is independent of religion, requires no belief in any deity, and is free of any reliance on sacred texts or authoritative teachers. It is based on reasoned argument. Philosophers, in other words, "do" ethics without religion. In the Roman Catholic tradition, the natural law approach has dominated ethical thinking, and it is essentially a philosophical approach based on the trust that God has given all people the potential for good will and reason. So, Catholics also "do" ethics in a manner that is more or less independent of the beliefs of the Catholic Christian faith.[2] Thus, people of all faiths and of no faith can engage in philosophical ethics, and so, in this sense, religion and ethics are distinct.

In another sense, however, the notion that all ethics is religious is true. Any system of ethical theory, although based on reason, requires some basic premises. Pure reason has no content. One cannot reason about morality without having a starting point from which to begin the process. These starting premises are incredibly difficult to prove, but they are necessary even for a philosophical system of ethics. In fact, most of the time, these premises are simply accepted through the exercise of a kind of "faith." These fundamental premises often contain a great deal of moral meaning. They express certain axiomatic (or near-axiomatic) beliefs about the meaning of life, death, good, evil, and human nature. If not frankly religious, these beliefs are at least "religion-like." In this sense, one can say that "every ethos implies a mythos."[3] Whether one begins in the "state of nature" or the "original position" or the "Garden of Eden," one must begin somewhere. Every ethical theory has some originating myth that has a religion-like character. Perhaps this explains why, when asked about the spiritual, some people immediately leap to the ethical.

Another reason clinicians tend to conflate the spiritual with the ethical may be that because it has been so hard for ethics to establish a beachhead in the medical arena, it is simply easier to try to line up spirituality behind the banner of ethics than to try to open a second front for spirituality. A strong minority within the medical community has persistently resisted such things as teaching ethics to students and residents, establishing ethics committees in hospitals (or cooperating with them where they exist), and enforcing codes of ethical conduct for practicing physicians and medical investigators. Organizational, procedural, and administrative resistance to allowing ethics a formal role in medicine has been common in both the academic and the practice communities. There has also been a degree of psychic resistance in the minds of some individual practitioners. In the minds of these physicians, ethics continues to be regarded as just one of those "soft" subjects. Proponents of spirituality in health care may simply believe that it is easier to lump spirituality in with ethics than to try to pick a new fight, dealing with spirituality on its own terms.

Perhaps, too, this conflation of the ethical and the spiritual represents something of a failure on the part of the various organized religions to make the distinction between spirituality and ethics clear to their members. At least this seems true of the Christian churches. Protestants, particularly fundamentalist Protestants, have always been suspicious of such spiritual practices as meditation, repetitive prayers, incense, icons, statues, and sacraments that characterize the mysticism of Catholic and Orthodox Christians. Instead, Protestants have emphasized scripture and the moral life. In the Catholic tradition since the Second Vatican Council, some of these traditional spiritual practices have been deemphasized in favor of a more psychologized approach to the inner life. This occurred along with a widespread questioning of traditional ethical teaching undertaken by some theologians, followed by a rather emphatic restatement of those traditional ethical teachings and an insistence on obedience on the part of the church. Many of these disputed ethical teachings touch on medicine. In such an environment, Catholicism has perhaps become overidentified with its ethical teaching and less identified with its spiritual practices. And this may help to explain why some clinicians conflate the spiritual with the ethical.

Last, in secularized Western societies, where people of many faiths and of no faith meet and interact daily, the moral life is a common ground of interaction among many diverse people. In such an environment, it seems that religions have sought to participate in society by emphasizing their contribution to ethical discourse. Religions "fit in" better when they are talking about ethics—the ethics of social justice, war and peace, science, and medicine. This is more acceptable in the public square than speaking frankly about prayer, spiritual experience, worship, the Buddha, or Jesus Christ. This "despiritualizing" of religion has also been turned inward within believing communities. In a sincere effort to be "relevant" to congregations that have become increasingly secularized through the overwhelming power of mass media, religions have tended to deemphasize the spiritual and have instead emphasized the ethical in their preaching. This may also partly explain why clinicians seem immediately to think "ethics" when they hear the word "spiritual."

The Spiritual

But the spiritual aspects of health care cannot be supplanted by bioethics. Hospitals, outside of the obstetric wards, are not usually happy places. As one walks down the corridors early in the morning on arrival at work, half awake, most of the other people one sees are fellow employees. Sometimes, however, one encounters a stranger—the woman without an identification badge, dressed not in scrubs but in a rumpled dress, walking slowly down the hall, her features barely discernible in the dim fluorescent light, biting her lip, fighting back the tears.

Did she just lose a husband? A mother? A son? Perhaps she was just told she has multiple sclerosis or cancer of the pancreas.

In the hospital the best it generally gets is relief—relief that the chest pain one experienced was not a heart attack; that one's prematurely born daughter, now on a ventilator, is likely to survive her harrowing first ninety days of life. Suffering shadows the work of health care professionals—a pervasive, profound, and persistent presence.

If health care professionals were honest, they would admit that they are just like most of the rest of secular society. They avoid eye contact. They demur at the thought of explicitly acknowledging suffering or their failure to make it all go away. They just keep walking.

If one is a Christian health care professional, however, one denies one's own creed by doing so. Sunday after Sunday Catholic Christians recite by rote, "He suffered, died, and was buried." If Christian health care professionals really knew Christ or understood what Christianity asks them to believe, they would understand immediately and intimately the spiritual dimension of their work that stares them in the face. Spirituality is not an ethical dilemma. It is the substance of what health care professionals do.

He suffered, died, and was buried. Just as our patients suffer, die, and are buried. Just as we suffer, die, and are buried. Ethics can make no sense of this. The way health care professionals behave in response to the reality of suffering may raise plenty of questions for ethics. But ethics itself will not help them to see their way through this. They can walk away. But the spiritual will be there again the next morning. In the corridor. Weeping.

Spirituality and Ethics

Simply put, spirituality describes one's relationship with the transcendent. Ethics, by contrast, can be defined as the systematic, critical, reasoned evaluation and justification of one's notions of right and wrong, good and evil, and of the kind of person one ought or ought not strive to become. By definition, these would appear to be quite distinct concepts. What, then, is the relationship between these two?

To answer this question, I must first make a further distinction between ethics and morality. Although these two words are often used interchangeably, ethics is, in a very formal way, the *study* of morality. Morality is the actual living, discerning, and doing of right and wrong, good and evil, and the actuality of either being or not being the kind of person one ought to be. Ethics is the effort to explain morality. But morality is where we live as human beings.

Thus understood, spirituality has much more to do with morality than it does with ethics (although trying to explain the relationship between morality and spirituality is an exercise in ethics). Spirituality is to theology as morality is to ethics. Human beings, by virtue of being the kinds of things that they are, are both spiritual and moral. One lives a human life as a spiritual and moral being. Explaining the spiritual and moral dimensions of human life are the tasks, respectively, of the disciplines of theology and ethics.

The good is known in the moral life in its individual instances— Mary's good and John's good. There is certainly a universal aspect to this good, depending, as it does, on the fact that both John and Mary are individual examples of the same kind of thing, that is, that both are human beings. What is good for each depends in large part on this fact. But one cannot promote the good of humankind concretely. One can only promote the good of John, or the good of Mary, or perhaps the good of their community. In the clinical world, this concrete good is the good of each particular patient. The health care practitioner has sworn to promote the good of particular patients.

Likewise, what is right is known in the moral life only in its individual instances—the right decision to forgo cardiopulmonary resuscitation or the right decision to build extra safety features into a research protocol, for example. Again, this is not to deny that some things are right and wrong for everyone. Establishing such principles is the task of ethics. But in the moral life, we decide what we think is right by making particular decisions in particular circumstances.

Yet the good and the right also have a transcendent dimension. Metaphorically speaking, the good and the right are the "wormholes" by which the parallel universes of the moral and the spiritual communicate. The person who is spiritually alive affirms that there is a Good beyond the sum of the good of each person and a Right beyond the sum of all morally correct decisions. The Good beyond all good and the Right beyond all right are not the abstract notions of good and right in ethical theory. Neither should this Good and this Right be identified with Platonic forms. I am invoking, instead, the moral horizon. Finitude and concreteness characterize human life, and these features of life are so explicit in the health care setting that clinicians and patients come to the brink of their deepest desires: Is there any meaning that is absolute? Any goodness that is infinite? Any relationship that is perfectly harmonious? Are there actual answers to these questions anywhere in the space and time of the universe or beyond it? To accept the possibility that these transcendent questions have an affirmative transcendent answer is to understand, in the first instance, how the spiritual passes over into the moral and the moral passes over into the spiritual.

The Numinous and the Medical

Rudolf Otto, in *The Idea of the Holy*, called the direct experience of transcendence an experience of the "numinous."[4] He invoked the notion of the *mysterium tremendum*—the apprehension of the transcendent, holy, and wholly other.[5] The numinous, as Otto pointed out, cannot be reduced to the morally good. The experience of the numinous is the experience of the awesome mystery that is so beyond human telling that it is what makes goodness good; it is an experience of goodness so vast and powerful that we shudder in shame, acutely conscious of our humanity and moral fallibility. Human beings have been describing such experiences for millennia and have named these as experiences of the divine. Such experiences most often occur in special times and places—on mountaintops, in religious shrines, on watching one's wife give birth, in meditation, while reading sacred scripture, while pondering a particularly profound theological work, or during a liturgy. These are the "oceanic" experiences of eternity and oneness with the universe that Freud deemed illusions and massive collective neuroses.[6] Freud denied that he had ever had such experiences, but it is my guess that he (the father of the theory of psychological repression), like many people, merely repressed his experiences. As the poet T. S. Eliot said, "We had the experience but missed the meaning."[7]

Such experiences are natural to humans. Human beings live their lives in relation to the infinite. We know the infinite reach of our desire. As Luigi Guissani put it, one must therefore either affirm oneself infinitely or affirm for oneself the infinite.[8] If one is sufficiently self-aware that one understands one's own finitude, only the latter makes sense. Put more simply, it has been said that Alcoholics Anonymous really has only two spiritual rules: (1) there is a higher power, and (2) you are not it.[9] These are the starting points of a spiritually informed moral life.

A Good Friday

The following is but one example of how spiritual experience can happen for a clinician. Once, during Holy Week, I attended the Good Friday liturgy at St. Francis of Assisi Church in New York City, where I was living at the time. I was thinking no particular thought, simply trying to be present to the Word of God proclaimed in my hearing; to the simple actions of procession, prostration, veneration; and to the sound of the organ and the smell of the incense. My gaze turned to the San Damiano crucifix in our church. This crucifix is a reproduction of the one from which Christ spoke to St. Francis in the ruined chapel of San Damiano. It is Byzantine in style. Although this image of the Crucified is very familiar to me, I noticed consciously for the first time that the belly of the Christ depicted on this crucifix is, oddly, a bit protuberant. My thoughts drifted, and I began to wonder why. Perhaps it was the artist's way of depicting Jesus's slumping body. Perhaps it was symbolic, meant to represent spiritual fecundity. Perhaps the artist just was not very good. Suddenly, however, another thought entered my mind. I saw there the protuberant belly of a patient I had seen the day before—a hospice nurse with a belly distended by cancerous fluid, a woman otherwise gaunt, obviously ill, and in profound denial, who had continued to work with hospice patients up to two weeks before her own hospitalization. She had told me of her eclectic background— ethnically Irish, English born, raised as an Anglican, and, on moving to New York, regularly attending both Episcopal church services and a Buddhist meditation group. She was unmarried and seemed very much alone in the world. She had attributed her sixty-pound weight loss, jaundice, swollen abdomen, troubled breathing, and rock-hard liver to "working too hard." The Passion narrative was being proclaimed from the pulpit, and my daydream and the Gospel intersected as I heard the cry from the cross, "My God, my God, why have you forsaken me?" In the painful site of this woman's thoracentesis (where a needle had been inserted to draw out fluid from around her right lung), I saw the lance that pierced the body of Christ on that same side. In her complaints about her dry mouth, I heard the words of Christ, "I thirst." I came to understand the Liturgy of the Passion in a profound way that day. And I wept as the numinous touched me. Overwhelmed me. Loved me.

Experiences like this one happen to everyone who is receptive to God's call—to all who live with eyes and ears and hearts that are open. These experiences are not illusions. They are glimpses into the deeper reality that makes sense of what we otherwise do. Such experiences can unite and sacramentalize an otherwise fragmentary world, connecting the woman biting her lip and walking slowly down the hospital corridor with the nurse dying of ovarian cancer. One finds that one is not far from any of these persons. All can be found in the belly of the crucified Christ.

These experiences come as gifts, in times and places not of human choice. One may prepare oneself for such experiences, but one may never conjure such experiences. They happen as naturally for health care professionals as they do for anyone else. They may happen often or infrequently. They happen with powerful intensity and with lesser intensity. They happen in different settings for different people and sometimes in different settings for the same person. But I am convinced that they happen for everyone.

Nonetheless, there is always a danger, especially in the twenty-first-century Western world, that one may clutter one's life in such a way as to dull one's spiritual senses to God's call. This is a particularly perilous professional liability in health care. This is how one may have the experience but miss the meaning. Classically, the only way to avoid this pitfall and keep one's spiritual senses sharp is through prayer.

Contemplation and Action

Prayer changes things. Most important, prayer changes the pray-er. After the Transfiguration experience, Peter, John, and James were initially seized with fear. They had glimpsed, for a moment, the *mysterium tremendum* in Jesus. They wanted to set up tents and stay on the mountain. But Jesus showed them why they could not remain there if they were to be his disciples. Immediately after descending the mountain, Jesus healed a possessed boy. He showed how prayer and praxis are connected. Contemplation leads to transformation, and transformation leads to loving action. Genuine contemplation is the wormhole through which the parallel universes of the spiritual and the moral communicate. When the disciples asked Jesus why they had been un-successful in their initial attempts at healing the same boy, he answered simply, "This kind can come out only through prayer" (Mk 9:29). That should be a lesson not just for the disciples but for all who practice the healing arts.

Grace is God's free gift of divine life to us. It can happen through prayer or meditation or spiritual disciplines or sacred reading or when we least expect it. Grace happens. Grace flows through the wormhole.

Grace acts on moral agents. Moral agents, in turn, act on the world. It is by God's grace alone that anyone who claims to be a healer ever said *honestly* to any admissions director of any professional school, "I want to help people."

Grace is the substance of religious motivation. Grace moved Albert Schweitzer from his comfortable life as a theologian and organist to medical school and eventually to his work in Africa. Grace moved Mother Teresa from Albania to India—first to a classroom and eventu-ally to the streets of Calcutta. Grace can move any physician or nurse from apathy to empathy; from discouragement to zeal; from self-absorption to conversion.

The numinous moves us. To experience, for as little as a moment, God's overwhelming love; to experience, for just a few passing minutes, the profound gratitude that all of us know, as rational creatures, ought to form the infrastructure of our lives; to be touched, if only for a sec-ond, by the mystery that holds everything in being—to experience these things requires a response. It is simply impossible to experience God in such a real way and not be moved to respond. And the only response that makes any sense is love.

This does not mean, of course, that our responses will be perfect. We are fallible, fragile, finite creatures. But the only way to try to avoid God's grace is to flee from it, to clutter one's life so that grace finds no room for expression, to bury it under mounds of ungodly pursuits, to distract one's attention from it by overemphasizing work or sexual plea-sure, to cloud one's ability to sense it with the use of mind-altering substances, or to rationalize it away with a complex set of witticisms designed to keep oneself alienated from one's own originating life force. Such evasive maneuvers will never work completely. Nonethe-less, one can shun God's grace enough to reduce oneself to such a weak state that one does not have the wherewithal to react to God's love with love. Sadly, such a state is perhaps more common among physicians than other persons in contemporary society.

One must be aware that one can also pervert religion, using it in such a way that it becomes a distraction from God—a means of alienating oneself from God. Persons who pervert religion in the name of morality fall broadly into two main types. Both give the appearance of being religious but are actually very busy keeping God as far away as possible. One type is the angry, nasty, judgmental, hyperorthodox type who finds heresy everywhere. The other type is the sly, slick, supercilious religious intellectual whose nuanced understanding of God is but an anemic projection of personal ego offered as a substitute for the transcendent, holy, loving, mysterious Other. Both types have become very common in the contemporary church. One feature they have in common is that both have reduced the spiritual to the moral. Thus, they often have much to say about issues in medical ethics. But they deserve far less attention than they now command in their polarizing styles. In the end, both types have affirmed themselves infinitely rather than affirming the infinite for themselves. Both seem to fear the one thing that could save them—surrender to the Mystery of God. A spiritual life reduced to a fixation with morality, whether devoted to twisting the moral rules to accommodate one's lifestyle or devoted to enforcing the moral rules tenaciously beyond the bounds of prudence, is no longer a Christian life. Only in the Mystery of God, made known in Jesus Christ, can the Good be apprehended and lived.

Practical Spirituality for Professionals

The rhythm of prayer and healing that informed the public life of Jesus Christ forms the perfect pattern for the Christian healer to emulate. Prayer is the opening of one's whole self to God. Between the "peak" experiences of the numinous, one must translate those experiences into daily life—at work and at home. One must continue to cultivate one's spirit, to let God speak not just on the mountaintop but also in the public square. In the public square of medicine, God tugs at the hem of one's white coat and asks for healing. One must cultivate the ability to sense when power goes out from one's own body and others are healed (Lk 8:46). Most clinicians remain blithely unaware.

To heal is to restore the state of right relations in a whole person. A healer whose own relations are set right is naturally in a better position to heal. One starts with one's own spirituality, one's own relationship with the transcendent, one's own experience of the Numinous One. To be an effective healer requires the true self-knowledge that comes only from a spiritual source. "What a person is before God, that he is, and no more," say the Admonitions of St. Francis.[10] Once one knows who one is in relationship to God, all other relationships fall more easily into place, including one's relationships with patients.

The ways one can accomplish this self-knowledge, even in the busy life of a clinician, are actually many and varied. One may prefer journaling, centering prayer, the rosary, Christian yogic meditation, *lectio divina* (a slow, contemplative method of reading scripture), or something else. The exact method is less important than the committed, intentional act. Busy people might also benefit by learning to become "opportunistic" pray-ers. What I mean by this is that one can take advantage of situations such as commuting (whether by public transportation or personal automobile) and learn to turn the delays and breakdowns into moments of prayer. Traffic jams can be transformed into graced moments with God rather than occasions of road rage. One need not spend all one's commuting time listening to Continuing Medical Education tapes. Dictating office notes while driving can be dangerous. Why not pray instead?

Although God can certainly appear when least expected, one can commit oneself to habitual practices of prayer that predispose one to hearing God's voice. One can prayerfully remember patients at the end of the day or cultivate a reverent mindfulness in one's daily practice. But whatever way one prays, it is important that one's practice inform one's spirituality every bit as much as one's spirituality ought to inform one's practice. That is the rhythm of Christian contemplation and action.

The transcendent questions of meaning, value, and relationship that are the fundamental questions of spirituality are visible everywhere in one's practice—provided one's eyes have been opened, and one has learned how to see. The transcendent can be found in the simple and the mundane.

For example, a twenty-four-year-old graduate student may show up as a walk-in to the office with a chief complaint of a new spot on her skin. She might say, "I've got this spot. It's been growing. Yesterday a friend saw it and said it looked like ringworm. I said it couldn't be ringworm. I mean, I take a bath every day. I'm a clean person."

One's temptation as a clinician is to the supercilious—to delight in one's superior knowledge and in the patient's ignorance. The physician knows this is not a hygiene problem. But the patient was truly troubled, in a simple way, by the *meaning* of what had befallen her. She was asking, indirectly, "Does this mean I'm dirty?"

She was also presenting with genuine questions of value: "What must people think of me now that I have this dirty disease?" She was also presenting with genuine questions of relationship: "Is this contagious? Can my boyfriend get it?"

And small as her problem might be, small as her questions might be, the ultimate term of each of these questions is transcendent. Health care professionals simply subsume it all under the name of the disease, *tinea corporis*, a fungal infection of the skin of the trunk.

But the routine ought never be boring in health care. The mundane is never far from the transcendent in the healing arts. Health care is the care of persons—beings in relationship with the transcendent. Clinicians are privileged to experience persons intimately in a fantastic, rich, multidimensional fashion.

When I saw this patient, I saw what she did not see. I saw a one-centimeter, somewhat hyperpigmented macule with a slightly raised and reddish edge located on her anterior left shin. I saw a dermatophyte infection. She saw "I am dirty." I saw her seeing "I am dirty."

Yet the healing commenced immediately, subtly, in a well-choreographed and well-rehearsed ritual. "No, it's not a parasite. It's a fungus. It's very common. Even people who bathe five times a day can get it." ("No, you are not dirty.")

"We can fix it easily. It will take time, but we're glad you came to see us today because we're catching it rather early. Come back in a month if it's not better." ("You are of value.")

"No, it's not contagious. Your boyfriend need not worry. No one at work need worry." ("Your relationships can be restored to normal. You will not die socially or physically. Not now. Someday, but not now.")

"Take this cream." ("Trust me. Enter into this relationship. You will be restored.")

Ten minutes. Bread-and-butter medicine. As mundane as it comes. But if God was not there, God is nowhere.

Grace and Virtue

The virtues are habitual predispositions to practices that express human excellence. The medical virtues include, among others, competence, compassion, patience, practical wisdom, and trustworthiness. Grace often intersects the life of a clinician in the realm of virtue. Grace motivates action in accord with virtue, and the more one acts virtuously, the more habitual it becomes, and the more it becomes characteristic of one's way of being in the world. Grace strengthens the hold of virtue—helps a person to maintain virtue in the face of challenges. Grace animates moral discernment—helps one to find and to maintain the proper balance of reason and affect, interpersonal proximity and distance, respect for life and acknowledgment of life's finitude. Medicine presents a challenging series of discernments each day. The work of health care, as a moral enterprise, demands virtue. The grace of God works efficaciously through virtue.

Clinicians need virtue. They need strength of character to ensure that the day-in and day-out practice of medicine never becomes drudgery. They need virtue to be lifelong learners, to know what they do not know, to accept the foibles of the patient as well as their own. They need to discern what is wrong, what can be done, and what ought to be done in the particular circumstances of the patients who come to see them.[11] These discernments are what make medicine an inherently moral enterprise. The process of moral discernment is a way of seeing—ultimately, a way of seeing the world as the world is seen by God. For a physician or nurse just once to see a patient as God sees her or him would be a graced moment indeed.

CHAPTER 2

Letter to a Young Intern

MEDICAL students, residents, and practicing physicians sometimes begin from a position of skepticism about spirituality and health care. One of many explanations for such skepticism is a set of deep, scarcely conscious, background presuppositions about the relationship between medical practice and outcomes that dominates the atmosphere of medicine today. This unconscious presupposition is that medicine is exclusively about outcomes. Cardiology researchers sometimes refer to this as the "body count," that is, that what really matters in medical research are the outcomes of clinical trials as measured in a "hard" number, such as mortality. Even "intermediary" outcomes, such as frequency of anginal symptoms or improved quality of life, are regarded as less valuable, less measurable, or "soft."

I do not wish to suggest that medicine should not be concerned with outcomes or that genuine spirituality is indifferent to outcomes. On the contrary, all physicians want to heal their patients, and well they should. Many spiritually enlightened persons (such as Jesus himself) have been great healers. But in the end, the really final outcome for all patients is metaphysically certain. All patients will die. Therefore, medicine cannot merely be about the outcomes. If it were, the whole enterprise would be futile at worst or trivial at best—just delaying the inevitable. Yet in medical discourse, one hears of almost nothing else but outcomes these days.

The idea that only outcomes count has been reinforced and even amplified by the spirit of American pragmatism, by the language and techniques of Total Quality Management (the latest fashion in hospital management), and even by the Evidence-Based Medicine movement.

This set of implicit background assumptions about medicine represents a more profound barrier to the introduction of spirituality into medical education and practice than is sometimes realized. To illustrate this, I have taken literary license and adapted a letter of Thomas Merton to the present situation in medicine.[1] I call this piece "Letter to a Young Intern." I share it as an example of how one might go about "doing" spirituality in a teaching hospital from the perspective of Christian spirituality. Regardless of the reader's own faith or lack of it, if one reads this piece as a clinician, the clash in perspective between professional discourse and this little meditation can serve to make those background assumptions explicit. This, in turn, may serve as a measuring rod for how difficult it will be to develop a real spirituality of health care in the twenty-first century. But at least the project will begin from a genuinely spiritual position.

LETTER TO A YOUNG INTERN (AFTER THOMAS MERTON)

Do not depend on the hope of results. When you are doing the work of health care, essentially an apostolic work, you may have to face the fact that your work will often be apparently worthless, and even achieve no result at all, if not perhaps results opposite to what you expect. As you get used to this idea, you start more and more to concentrate not on the results but on the value, the truth of the work itself.

And there, too, a great deal has to be gone through, as gradually you struggle less and less for some scientific ideal and more and more for specific patients. The range tends to narrow down but it gets much more real. In the end, it is the reality of personal relationships that saves everything.

You are fed up with all this talk about outcomes, and I do not blame you. I am nauseated by it sometimes. I am also, to tell the truth, nauseated by total quality management and evidence-based medicine. This sounds like heresy, but I think you will understand what I mean. It is easy to become so completely engrossed with Southern blots and odds ratios and randomized controlled trials that in the end one is left alone in the denouement of an unsuccessful code, tangled in a web of electrocardiogram tracings, holding the Ambu bag, empty, with no trace of meaning left in it. The temptation sets in to yell louder than ever in order to make the meaning be there again by some form of scientific operation. But it does not work. Going through this kind of reaction at least once may help you to guard against all sorts of spiritual dangers. Your system is complaining of too much emphasis on outcomes, and it is right.

You know all too well that the big results are not in your hands or mine. Good clinical outcomes seem big, but their greatness diminishes with the passing of time. And those really great clinical moments are rare enough. They happen suddenly, and we can experience great joy in them, like the moment of profound satisfaction that comes in making a rapid and correct diagnosis of meningitis and having it confirmed by the laboratory hours after you have already started the antibiotics. And, wonder of it all, the patient may actually live to thank you. You think to yourself, "This is what I went to school for." You are overwhelmed, just for a moment, with justified pride and for a few seconds even have a glimpse beyond yourself and your patient toward something far more significant. But there is no point in any of us building our lives on such moments, which may be denied us by failed experiments or unsuccessful operations or by angry or ungrateful patients. After all, this sort of professional satisfaction is really not that important.

The next step in the process is for you to see that it is your own thinking about what you are doing that is crucially important. I will bet that you are probably striving to build yourself an identity in your work, out of your work and the recognition of others. You are using it, so to speak, to protect yourself against nothingness, annihilation. That is not the right use of your work. All the good that you will do will come not from you but from the fact that you have allowed yourself, in the obedience of faith, to be used by God's love. Think of this more, and gradually you will be free of the need to prove yourself, and you can be more open to the power that will work through you without your knowing it.

The great thing, after all, is to live, not to pour out your life in the service of a scientific theory; and we turn the best things, even spirituality, into scientific theories. If you can get yourself free of the domination of outcomes and just serve Christ's truth, you will actually find that you are able to do more, and you will be less crushed by the inevitable disappointments—such as those occasioned by the kindly old man with lymphoma who suddenly "crashes" and dies; or by the patient with diabetes who repeatedly stops taking her insulin and returns over and over again to the emergency room in diabetic ketoacidosis; or by the rejection of a paper submitted to the *New England Journal of Medicine*.

Every career in medicine will inevitably be marked by its share of disappointment, frustration, and confusion. The real hope, then, is not in something we think we can do, but in God, who is making something good out of it in some way we cannot see. If we can do God's will, we will be helping out in the process. But we will not necessarily know about it all beforehand.

I hope this makes some sense to you. You may be too young to understand, but you will be a better doctor the moment you do. Can you bring yourself to realize that the patient's outcome is really none of your business? Now that's a scary thought. I wouldn't advise that you tell the Chief of Medicine just yet . . .

Catholic Christianity and the Meaning of Healing

*I*N this chapter I explore the meaning of healing from the perspective of Catholic Christianity. What I propose is not completely unique to Catholic Christianity. In fact, I hope it resonates deeply with persons of other religious traditions. Yet, there are different emphases and shadings that will inevitably impart a distinctive approach to spirituality and health care within any particular tradition. This may be especially true of Catholicism. Accordingly, my approach will be both descriptive and constructive. I will describe features that have characterized a Catholic approach to health care, but I will also suggest some new ways of conceiving the meaning of healing that grows out of that tradition. Monks and sisters and committed lay health care professionals have lived lives of service to the sick in ways that are distinctively Catholic for centuries, and some have written a few words about how they have found God among the sick. To the best of my knowledge, however, no one has tried to ask before what healing means in the Catholic tradition. That meaning, I hope, will have broad implications for all persons who are seriously interested in spirituality and health care.

It seems indisputable that healing has played a major role in the lived experience of Christian faith from the beginning. Yet Roman Catholic Christianity has placed an emphasis on healing that is perhaps distinctive among the Christian churches. Healing is woven into the fabric of the Catholic Church's spiritual, sacramental, and ministerial life. All Christians pray for the sick. Certainly, other Christian churches have healing services. Miraculous physical healings seem

central, for instance, to American Protestant Revivalist prayer meetings. But only Catholics and Orthodox Christians have a *Sacrament* of
the Sick. Other Christian churches have embraced health care as a
ministry, and some have even sponsored hospitals, but none to the extent that Catholics have done so. For example, the first modern physicians were medieval monk-herbalists. And even today, 16 percent of
the hospital admissions in the United States are to facilities operated
under Catholic auspices.[1]

So, what does healing mean in Catholic consciousness that makes
it so important? Ironically, despite all the distinctively Catholic emphasis on religious practice and healing, I think the Catholic understanding of the meaning of healing is more generically Christian than
specifically Catholic. Because I think the Catholic answer to the question will be based largely on what Jesus said and did as recorded in
scripture, it is an answer that any Protestant Christian could easily give.
Obviously, there are also aspects of the Catholic answer that will reso-
nate vibrantly with other systems of religious belief. In the end, what
makes Catholic healing *Catholic* is not a different belief about what
healing means but rather the way this church has given shape to the
Christian meaning of healing in a typically Catholic, Incarnational
fashion. That is to say, Catholics have shaped the meaning of Christian
healing in the very concrete, in-the-flesh ways that characterize the
Catholic Christian tradition.

Catholics give expression to Christian healing in three distinctive
ways. First, Catholics emphasize seeing God in the book of nature as
well as in the book of scripture: Catholics tend to see God in the nature
of their own concrete experiences with illness and healing. It is therefore no accident that the stories of the great saints of the Catholic faith
are quite often stories of conversion through the experience of illness
or injury. Second, Catholics express their faith in concrete forms that
they call sacraments and so express the meaning and importance of
healing in sacramental ways. For example, not only is there a Sacrament of the Sick but also before every communion Catholics echo the
words of the centurion seeking healing for his servant and say, "Only
say the word and I shall be healed." And, finally, Catholics have a
tendency to create institutions, enshrining their ministries in bricks
and mortar. If Catholics consider something a genuine ministry, Catholics will build a home for it. And so it is no accident that there are so
many Catholic hospitals.

But the Catholic expression of the meaning of Christian healing is not the meaning itself. In the rest of this chapter, I will offer a more fundamental reflection on the meaning of healing. I would like to suggest that Christian healing can be understood in three important ways—as the restoration of right relationships, as encounter, and as witness.

Healing as the Restoration of Right Relationships

Many spiritually minded persons take healing, based on its etymology, to mean "making whole." Claims like this are not uncommon. But what does this "making whole" really mean? All too often, the understanding of "making whole" is quite facile, leading to very loose talk about "holistic" health care. Certainly, one cannot be opposed to "holistic" care if this means attentiveness to the ill person's psychosocial and spiritual needs. "Holistic," however, sometimes includes the most banal fringes of New Age spirituality, suggesting, almost, that immortality can be achieved through dietary manipulation. I believe healing *is* a making whole, but in a very particular way.

The understanding of healing that I would like to offer, however, first requires taking a step back from health care. At the risk of seeming grandiose, I want to suggest that to understand the meaning of healing in the new way I am proposing requires one to understand the constitution of the universe itself in a way that might at first seem unfamiliar and strange.

A complete explication of what I am proposing would require a much longer discourse in physics and metaphysics than is possible in a limited number of pages. But briefly, the understanding I would like to share, emerging largely from contemporary physics, is this: That the most basic stuff of the universe, the stuff we call matter, can no longer be understood as merely what remains after chopping up physical bodies into smaller and smaller parts. "Chopping" is what physics, biology, and medicine did so successfully until the twentieth century—breaking up bodies into parts, parts into molecules, molecules into atoms, and atoms into subatomic particles. But once one arrives at the particle level, a fundamental rule emerges that is really true about everything, no matter how big or small, namely, that relationality is ontologically prior to particularity, that the electromagnetic field is prior to matter.

That is to say that what matter, or anything else, is, at its most fundamental level, is not a pile of unimaginably tiny bodies, but a set of temporary yet dynamic relationships in the electromagnetic field that is already given. Subatomic particles, the so-called building blocks of matter itself, can only be understood as entities defined by complex relationships. As physicist Niels Bohr once put it, "In our description of nature the purpose is not to disclose the real essence of the phenomena but only to track down, so far as it is possible, relations between the manifold aspects of our experience."[2] The naïve atomism of Democritus, smashed by Aristotle, revived again by Galileo, refined by Dalton, and made normative by Mill, has been smashed again by Einstein, Planck, Bohr, and Heisenberg. Matter is not isolated bits of individual particularity. Matter itself is relational.

From a philosophical point of view, as Bernard Lonergan has argued, when one knows some "thing" (literally, any "thing"), what one is really grasping is a complex set of relationships, whether that thing is a quark, a virus, a patient, or a galaxy.[3] In a few brief pages I cannot say more, but the take-home message is this: being *is* relationship.

For the Christian, this truth is preeminently understood as the very nature of the Triune God. God *is* a relationship: Father, Son, and Spirit.

Less obviously, sickness, rightly understood, is a disruption of right relationships. It is not "looking at a bad body inside an otherwise healthy body." As Frank Davidoff has asked, "Who has seen a blood sugar?"[4] Diabetes is not a "bad body" that one sees through the lens of some device, but a disturbance in that set of right relationships that constitutes the homeostasis of the thing we call a human being.

Ancient peoples readily understood sickness as a disturbance in relationships. Because these peoples had a keen sense of the relationship between human beings and the cosmos, the task of the shaman was to heal by restoring the relationship between the sick person and the cosmos. Thus, healing was a religious act. It consisted in the restoration of right relationships between people and their gods.

Contemporary scientific healing also consists in the restoration of right relationships. Nevertheless, scientific healing heretofore has understood this as limited to the restoration of those relationships that constitute the homeostasis of the patient as an individual organism. From a purely scientific point of view, healing means restoring the balance of blood sugar in relation to other biochemical processes; restoring the due regard cancer cells ought to have in relation to other cells; restoring the proper temporal relationship between the pacemaker cells of the heart and other physiological processes; restoring blood pressure to the level that allows the heart and lungs to maintain their proper relationships with the other vital organs.

But illness disturbs more than relationships *inside* the human organism. It disrupts families and workplaces. It shatters preexisting patterns of coping. It raises questions about one's relationship with God.

Jesus also understood healing as the restoration of right relationships in this fuller sense. I think that is why his healing miracles occur so often in association with reconciliation. Before he heals the paralytic, he says, "Your sins are forgiven" (Mt 9:1–8; Lk 15:17–26). When his own disciples question Jesus about the man born blind, they ask, "Whose sin caused his condition?" Jesus restores right relationships within the community as well as within the physiology of the man by declaring, as he heals him, that neither his sins nor his parents' sins caused the illness (Jn 9:1–40). Frequently, Jesus states as he heals, "Your faith has made you well" (Mk 10:52). The faith to which Jesus refers is relational. The faith associated with the healing miracles is not assent to the propositions of a creed but to a trusting relationship with Jesus. Before being healed the blind beggar must reach out to Jesus and say, "Son of David, Jesus, have pity on me" (Mk 10:47).

And Jesus frequently heals at the behest of the patient's *relations*. Thus, Jesus restores family relationships when he heals: for the widow who had lost her son (Lk 7:11–17); for Jairus, who was losing his daughter (Lk 8:40–42, 49–56); for Peter, whose mother-in-law was ill (Mt 8:14–15); for Martha and Mary, who had lost their brother Lazarus (Jn 11:1–44); and for the centurion whose household was losing a cherished servant (Mt 8:5–13).

What medicine seems to be missing today, and Christianity can help bring back to it, is this broad understanding of healing as the restoration of right relationships—not only relationships inside the body but also those between the sick and their families, their communities, and God.

Healing as Encounter

For the Christian, healing is also a direct encounter with God. I know of no other religious figure before Jesus who makes a claim as remarkable as the claim of Matthew 25, "I was sick and you came to visit me." In Christianity, visiting the sick and caring for their needs is not merely a moral duty, but an actual encounter with Christ. He says, "You came to visit *me*." The one who reaches out to the sick person finds God— and not just in the act of helping the person, but in the person himself or herself, because the sick person, according to the scriptures, is already Christ, waiting. The patient is thus an *alter Christus*, another Christ. If one really understands what this means, one will see that it is a theologically stunning claim.

To be a healer is to find God in those in need of healing. For the Christian, healing is a direct encounter with the divine. And that encounter, if genuine, necessarily causes personal transformation. In the parable of the Good Samaritan, the priest and the Levite ignore *God* when they ignore the wounded man, and so their lives remain unchanged—they keep walking down the same path (Lk 10:29–37). The man the Good Samaritan finds bleeding on the side of the road is really the Lord. And in picking him up and binding his wounds, the Samaritan's life is changed. Likewise, St. Bonaventure suggested that, in embracing the leper, St. Francis of Assisi embraced Christ himself, who, as Isaiah had prophesied (Is 53:3), was like a leper, outcast and despised.[5] After this encounter, the life of Francis was never the same again.

So, although religious health care professionals may often want to understand themselves as "channels" for God's healing power, Christianity teaches that they would perhaps be better served if they understood themselves first and foremost as persons privileged to serve God by serving the sick.

Healing as Witness

Jesus commissioned his disciples to "cure the sick," and this was clearly part of their charge to spread the "good news" of the Gospel (Mt 10:1, 7; Mk 16:18; Lk 9:1–6). So, while healing may be an encounter with God, there also appears to be a sense in which Christ intended that healing should be a way of evangelizing, of announcing that the reign of God is at hand. And the disciples clearly did this. The Acts of the Apostles records the many healings they performed in the name of Christ (Acts 3:1–10; 5:12–16; 9:36–43; 20:7–12).

But one might wonder why healing should be such a special sign of the presence of God. Christ himself could have performed other sorts of miracles and could have asked the disciples likewise to announce his presence by performing miracles that had nothing to do with healing. If the purpose of the miracles were only to show God's power, then why not turn the Temple into gold, make people fly, or turn stones into bread (Lk 4:3-4) or frogs into princes? True, there *is* the story of Jesus turning water into wine, but that was because his mother asked (Jn 2:1-11)! What else could a good Jewish boy like Jesus do under such circumstances? The vast majority of Jesus's miracles were miracles of healing, despite the fact that other actions would clearly have been just as convincing as displays of God's power.

It is perhaps also significant that miracles of healing are the predominant miracles of the New Covenant, not the Old Covenant. Although there are a few stories of miraculous healing in the Hebrew scriptures, such as Elisha healing Naaman the leper (2Kgs 5), Isaiah healing Hezekiah's boil (Is 38:21), and Tobias curing his father Tobit's blindness with the help of the angel Raphael (Tb 11:1-16), most of the miracles of the Old Covenant were of a different sort—burning bushes, parted seas, and pillars of fire. These are miracles of power and awe, not of healing.

Perhaps the vast majority of the miracles of the New Testament are miracles of healing because healing has particular features that make it especially suitable as the miracle of choice for Jesus and his disciples. One of the reasons that Jesus healed is that healing is evangelical. It is symbolic of the good news made manifest in Jesus. God's dream for the universe has always been, ever since the sin of Adam, the dream of universal reconciliation—the complete restoration of right relationship everywhere. Healing the body is thus, par excellence, a sign of God's reconciling love. Healing an individual's body announces the healing of the Mystical Body of Christ. The broken human family needs the homeostasis that God promises in Christ Jesus. Healing the body of any individual human being ought to remind that person of his or her radical dependence on God. Healing is never peripheral to who we are as embodied creatures. Such things as the creation of gold, heroic or unusual feats, and the acquisition of power or prestige are really peripheral to our humanity. Healing is about who we are as persons integrally considered, as finite embodied creatures made in God's own

image and likeness. And so healing is truly an evangelical act. It announces all this good news.

Christians heal because they are commanded by Christ to do so.
Healing is a special sign of God's promise of universal right relationship. And Christians do not heal by any power they possess, but by
virtue of their need to share with others the good news they have
heard, announced by and in Jesus.

Obviously, those who are nonbelievers can also heal. Much of medicine today, with its success (and also with its emptiness), is the healing
of unbelief. In a limited, technical sense, this kind of healing "works,"
but those who heal thinking that they have done so by their own power
commit the sin of Simon Magus, the magician from scripture who
asked the apostles for the power to confer the spirit on people through
the laying on of hands, even offering to pay them for it (Acts 8:9–25).
Too many health care professionals today do not understand that all
healing comes from God (Sir 38:1–15) and harbor the false belief that
healing is something they can buy, possess, or control. The moment
one grasps for it, the power to heal in the fullest sense of the word
disappears.

Likewise, many people are healed today and fail to recognize what
has happened to them in a deeper way. This is clearly true of most
patients in the Western world. This precise situation is described in the
Gospel story of Jesus's healing of ten lepers, only one of whom returns
to thank him. Perhaps nine out of ten lepers today, once healed, forget
to return to Jesus to thank him for having cured them. And so Jesus
inquires after all those patients who leave our hospitals today, having
considered cure their entitlement, "Why has only one returned to
thank me? Where are the other nine?" (Lk 17:11–19). Gratitude is the
right relationship between any healed human being and God. Gratitude announces the reign of the One who heals.

Conclusion

In this chapter I have sketched out three ways of understanding the
meaning of healing from a Catholic Christian perspective—as the restoration of right relationships, as encounter with Christ, and as witness
to Christ. All three happen simultaneously and inseparably every time
a physician, nurse, psychologist, or other health care professional

reaches out, in faith, to any one of God's children who is sick. Among our major tasks in health care today is to rediscover a form of practice that can heal the health care system in just the same way. Our health care system is sick, out of balance, and fraught with distorted and bizarre relationships. Yet even in a depersonalized system of care such as our own, those who can see their service to the sick as ministry may finally become humble enough to recognize that they are not God and respectful enough of their patients to recognize in them the face of the divine. And those who can do so will truly be able to announce by deeds that speak more loudly than words that the reign of God, God's dream of universal right relationship, is at hand.

CHAPTER 4

Appearance and Morality

MOST health care professionals genuinely strive for the good of their patients. That they do so even under today's difficult working conditions redounds to their credit. But if one is to resist attitudes that are so characteristic of the present era, one will want to know more about the meaning of the patient's good than the common assumption that it means only what the patient thinks is good for him or for her.

One often hears that working for the patient's good means attending to the patient's "values," and this suggestion is taken to be the surest way to escape the troubles caused by our overly technological approach to health care. Nevertheless, "values talk" really does not offer a path of liberation from technology. "Values talk" is actually better considered a *symptom* of the technological approach to health care. "Values talk" has emerged because technology has now completely encompassed all aspects of human life. In fact, it has been observed that "technology . . . is the unspoken and invisible framework of discussion of values."[1] "Values talk" actually represents the industrialization of morality. To elicit the patient's "values" and then attempt to engineer them into an "outcome" is an approach that is concerned almost exclusively with technique—a technology of ethics. To speak of "values" is not to speak of a moral alternative to technology, but to accept the usurpation of morality by technology. Policy analysis, decision analysis, and cost-benefit analysis are all industrial techniques that present themselves as complete ethical systems. Yet each of these is merely a technique for determining the most efficient way to maximize "values." In and of themselves these techniques provide no way to justify values or to judge them as good or bad. Technology in general "comes into play as the indispensable and unequalled procurement of the means that allow us realize our preferred values."[2] This holds whether the technology is a machine or a procedure for values clarification.

"Values," however, are not automatically good simply because they are preferred or chosen. One will not arrive at the patient's good merely by asking each for his or her values.

The religious approach to moral questions, and the approach favored over most of the history of Western philosophy up until the time of Nietzsche, did not prescribe the pursuit of the arbitrary values that people happen to have chosen as individuals. If one is to continue to make use of the contemporary word "values," serious ethics requires that one must specify the *right* values—the ones that are universal and apply to all people.

Plato thought that there were three such ultimate right values: Beauty, Truth, and Goodness. The great doctor of the church, St. Augustine of Hippo, agreed. Plato called these values "Forms." Augustine thought they were attributes of God.

The three ultimate right values of Plato and Augustine—Beauty, Truth, and Goodness—have more to do with health care than one might at first think. I want to argue that these are the ultimate right values of a health care professional's work—that the good of the patient subsists in these three ultimate right values. The professional world in which doctors, nurses, and other health care professionals work, day in and day out, is subsumed under the canopy of these three ultimate right values. The clinical decisions that health care professionals make every day involve the struggle to hold these ultimate values together, to balance them, to harmonize them, and to respect them.

I fully realize that most clinicians do not think themselves worthy of such a lofty discussion, but this may illustrate their relative lack of attention to the deep human significance of health care. Clinicians struggle to harmonize Beauty, Truth, and Goodness in and through the body in which these values literally take on human flesh. Persons speak, listen, touch, taste, write, play, love, and worship through their bodies.

Twenty-First-Century Confusion

Our society, however, deals with the values of Beauty, Truth, and Goodness in a confused and distorted fashion. In the end, this confusion has an impact on health care. Beauty is highly valued by contemporary society, but in an astonishingly superficial way. Fashion models and movie stars set standards of beauty and perpetual youth nearly impossible for anyone else to reach. Under this influence, charlatan physicians convince hordes of people (who want to be convinced) that a secret combination of vitamins and herbs combined with a regimen of leisure will guarantee a perpetually youthful face. Botox parties have supplanted Tupperware parties. And we are confronting an epidemic of eating disorders.

Truth is similarly distorted by contemporary society. Marketing strategy supplants and even scoffs at the notion of Truth. Manipulation supplants rational persuasion. "Spin" supplants the classical art of rhetoric. And this approach contaminates everything from dating to art to politics. Sadly, even among medical researchers the truth is bypassed all too often for the sake of fame or greed.

And Goodness? Taxpayers and insurance companies cannot seem to find enough of it to pay for medical care for the poor, the undocumented, or the more than forty million American citizens who are uninsured. The increasing consumerism of our society has distorted the very meaning of the Good. Rather than an ultimate right value for which everyone strives, the Good has become reduced to the pathetic little question, "What's in it for me?"

Morality and Practice

Yet each health care professional is called, by the nature of the practice, to a moral life that must transcend this pedestrian indifference to morality that governs so much of our society. Health care, by its very nature, is a moral enterprise.[3] The sick come to physicians and surgeons vulnerable, frightened, often shunned by others, and unable to help themselves. Physicians, surgeons, and other health care professionals have taken oaths by which they have sworn to help those who come to them in the predicament of illness or injury. Every time a patient walks into the examining room, and a clinician grasps that patient's hand and says, "Hi. I'm Dr. Jones. How can I help you?" a profound moral event occurs. A promise is made in that moment—that all the hard years of education and training and debt and delayed gratification have been fixed on the moment of need of *this* patient. In every patient encounter, each health care professional puts his or her oath (and very self) on the line.[4] Each renews that oath with each patient, one patient at a time. And in the end, no matter how much doctor shopping may have taken place before, finally, that patient has no choice but to trust that at least one clinician will be true to that promise.

The more vulnerable the patient, the less able to speak for himself or to get up and leave the office, the truer it is, but, in the end, each and every patient, no matter how old, no matter how small, no matter how ugly or deformed, whether wanted or unwanted by others, must trust that the doctors and nurses who care for that individual will be true to that promise. And if there are *any* patients for whom clinicians cannot be true to that promise, then we will never be able to trust that they will be true to that promise for the rest of us.

This recurring moral event—this recursive enactment of the oath—is made especially vivid when one cares for the deformed. Pedestrian amorality shuns the unattractive and the ugly. But many health care professionals confront it on a daily basis. Some may even be called on deliberately to *cause* it.

Clinicians sometimes need to be reminded that the ugly and the deformed are among the greatest social outcasts. In a classic survey, 77 percent of research subjects inferred from the description of a person as intelligent, industrious, warm, determined, practical, and cautious that the person must be good looking.[5] From childhood, people learn not to pity but to laugh at those who are not beautiful. Later in life, the homely and the deformed are passed over in job interviews. They have trouble finding love. No one wants to be seen with them at work or in social circles. The ugly and the deformed have always been among the greatest outcasts in any society, but perhaps never so much before as in our own media-saturated twenty-first century.

It is vital to avoid the trap of denying the reality of ugliness and deformity. Although it is true that all are beautiful in God's eyes, this attitude ought never become a pious veil that prevents us from seeing deformity and ugliness for what they are. Genuine Christian spirituality does not deny the existence of the ugly but affirms the paradoxical beauty that can only be known by resisting the temptation to avert one's eyes.

Consider especially the care of those who are deformed in the head or the face. In caring for such patients, one's professional gaze is fixed on the primary venue in which human beings relate to each other as persons. The head is the primary means by which people identify others and are in turn identified by them. To be convinced of this, one need only to recognize that a bust or a portrait is sufficient to represent an entire person. It is through our heads (and especially through our faces) that we encounter each other as persons. The head is the home of the face, the eyes, the voice, and the mind. Four of the five special senses belong exclusively to the head. Patients whose illnesses affect their heads and faces are therefore especially afflicted.

All clinicians confront ugliness and deformity in at least two ways. First, persons with deformities come to them for repair and restoration of their natural beauty, now ravaged by injury or disease: the healing of a rash, the repair of a congenital cleft palate, the repair of a saddle-nose deformity caused by the rare autoimmune disease Wegener's granulomatosis, or even the simple restoration of a normal voice by the prescription of drugs and the restitution of normal sinus drainage. Physicians, nurses, and other health care professionals can help to restore the natural beauty of persons others would shun. This is a truly awesome power and carries with it a profound moral responsibility.

But even more challenging are those cases in which clinicians must actually undertake procedures that *cause* deformity. An oncologist may be called on to give chemotherapy to a teenage girl, knowing that he will make her go bald and induce sores on her lips. A surgeon may be asked to take out the cancerous side of a person's face or to remove the orbit and sinuses of a person infected with mucormycosis, a potentially fatal fungal infection. How can this be? In the name of Beauty, Truth, and Goodness, by what authority might any person claim the right to do such things?

Beauty, Truth, and Goodness

This question brings me back to Plato and Augustine. In the *Symposium* (201–2), Plato argued that love is always love of the beautiful.[6] Love is a desire for a beauty one does not possess. But Plato argued further that although the Good and the True are always beautiful, what appears to be beautiful is not always good or true. Plato argued that the wise person loves beauty in its deeper sense—the beauty of Goodness and Truth. This beauty is the beauty of the *person*.

Clinicians come to know this beauty only by confronting ugliness squarely. A surgeon, for example, might come to understand this beauty only after the cold steel of surgical truth has laid bare the most hideous of lesions. For an oncologist, the terrible and fearful beauty of completely ablated bone marrow, viewed under a microscope, might very well be that kind of deep Platonic beauty. But one must have eyes trained to see it.

Of the aesthetics of the human body, and of this deeper human beauty, Augustine said:

> Now if it is true (and it is scarcely a matter for debate) that there is no visible part of the body which is merely adapted to its function without being also of aesthetic value, there are also parts which have only aesthetic value without any practical purpose. Hence it can, I think, be readily inferred that in the design of the human body dignity was a more important consideration than utility. For practical needs are, of course, transitory; and a time will come when we shall enjoy one another's beauty for itself alone.[7]

Pedestrian amorality often shuns the patients whom surgeons, physicians, nurses, psychiatrists, and other health care professionals are called on to serve. And their treatments are rarely perfectly restorative. Strive as mightily as a surgeon might to preserve form and function, the postsurgical voice still often sounds quite unnatural, the face not quite normal, the control of salivation not quite perfect. The bulging of exophthalmos (abnormally protruding eyes) may persist for a lifetime, despite the endocrinologist's success in cajoling Graves' disease into remission. But this need not be the final word on the patient's beauty. A clinician who is spiritually aware leads the way beyond pedestrian amorality to the higher ethic that his or her specialty demands. Plato said to those who would denigrate such work, "What blasphemy! Do you think that anything that is not beautiful must necessarily be ugly?"[8]

Still, one is required to confront the moral questions raised by the most extensive and aggressive treatments. Are there any that simply ought never to be done? Can one so deform a patient that, even though he or she might have a good prognosis for survival, the treatment ought not to be given even if requested by the patient?

For instance, consider the incredibly extensive and profoundly disfiguring operation known as hemicorporectomy (the removal of the whole lower part of the body, from the pelvis down), which has been performed on more than forty patients despite very low survival rates.[9] Even though the procedure can be accomplished successfully from a technical point of view, controversy still exists as to whether such surgery should be done at all. If that is true of the lower body, what might be true of radical treatments that will deform the head or face?

Several years ago I had the privilege of attending rounds with one of our head and neck surgeons at St. Vincent's, Dr. Jordan Stern. We saw a man who had undergone, at the patient's own insistence, a total surgical removal of the tongue and larynx for squamous cell cancer. As is often the case, his social supports were weak. He was homeless, living in a church basement. He was unemployed and had recently moved to New York from another state, leaving behind his wife and child, fleeing child support, and seeking Supplemental Security Income and Medicaid benefits. He had lived much of his adult life in a California hippie commune and had an extensive history of abusing drugs, alcohol, and tobacco. He stated that his diagnosis, which occurred shortly after he arrived in New York, had changed his life—that he had undergone a religious conversion and had given up his substance abuse. Yet this conversion had not convinced him of any obligations to his family. The patient had done remarkably well with surgery. His recovery was quick, and his extensive incisions were healing nicely. He seemed stunningly optimistic and happy for a man who had just been rendered unable to eat or speak, with a large scar and a high likelihood of dying nonetheless from his underlying disease. Considering the whole man, the immediate surgical result was far neater than the psychosocial milieu out of which the tumor arose and into which he was returning. Where are the Beauty, Truth, and Goodness in such a situation?

I think that answering this question requires that one understand how these three ultimate right values are related to each other. According to Plato, as I said above, Goodness and Truth are deeper than the mere appearance of beauty. But Plato further discerned that Goodness is deeper than Truth. As he put it in his *Republic* (508e), "Both knowledge and truth are beautiful, but you will be right to think of the Good as more beautiful than they."[10] Similarly, Augustine said, "Of all these goods, however, whether of soul or body, there is none at all that virtue puts above herself. For virtue makes good use of herself and all the other goods which bring man happiness. But if she herself is not there, then, however many goods there are, they do the possessor no good, and so are not to be called his 'goods.'"[11]

Knowing that Goodness and Truth supersede Beauty and that Goodness supersedes Truth does not constitute a simple algorithm for answering clinical questions. Ethics gives a compass, not an itinerary. But I will suggest that these ethical admonitions mean that virtuous clinicians, and all their patients, would be well served if, in all their clinical decision making, their ultimate value were always the good of the patient. Whatever truth one comes to acquire through research must serve the good of the patient. The truths of the patient's condition and prognosis have no point *but* to serve the good of the patient. The beauty one strives to restore in the patient's body must be for the good of the patient. And any beauty one forgoes for the sake of cure or palliation must be for the good of the patient. I do think there are some contemplated treatments for which the stark reality of the truth of the matter and the steep effacement of beauty are of such anticipated magnitude that such treatments could never truly serve the good of the patient as a person. For example, in a frontal lobotomy for refractory schizophrenia, in the hemicorporectomy described above, or in chest compressions on a person whose bones have been reduced to gristle by metastatic malignancy, survival, if it comes at all, would occur only at the cost of utter defacement. When one reaches this point, morality demands that one lay aside needle, knife, or scope and affirm for the patient that one understands this deeper beauty and will remain committed to serving his or her good. The beauty born of such a moment is tragic, but it is beautiful nonetheless, precisely because it is good and true.

Responsibility

In all one does as a health care professional, one must consider the remarkable moral responsibility that comes with this role. Clinicians are challenged daily to help men and women as they struggle to know what Beauty, Truth, and Goodness could possibly mean in the face of horrible illness. But more than this, the rest of society depends on health care professionals to show the way. Health care professionals must therefore be moral exemplars, teaching everyone else moral lessons that are very hard to learn. One lesson is that one must always bear in mind, in confronting the horrors that clinicians confront, one's own dependence on others and one's human solidarity with the one who is suffering. Once one understands this, figuring out what to do becomes infinitely easier. As the philosopher Alasdair MacIntyre put it, "Of the brain damaged, of those almost incapable of movement, of the autistic, of all such we have to say: this could have been us."[12] Against the all-too-human inclination to shrink from those to whom fate has dealt severe and even mortal blows, health care professionals must always act out of the moral stance, "It could have been me." Society must learn that lesson from its health care professionals. That is a profound responsibility. MacIntyre went on to say,

> Consider that kind of disablement which consists in gross disfigurement of the surface of body parts, perhaps of a swollen, inflamed, scarred, and secretion-exuding face, where the horrifying and disgusting appearance of the sufferer becomes an obstacle in addressing her or him as a human being. Nurses or physicians whose duty it is to understand the sufferer's appearance as a set of symptoms of an underlying condition have perhaps an easier task than the rest of us who need to find some way of avoiding both the mistakes involved in pretending that the sufferer does not, in fact, present an horrifying appearance, and those involved in being too distracted by that appearance to be able to deal rationally with the sufferer. What we may learn about ourselves from grappling with these difficulties is in part the nature and the degree of value that we have hitherto placed upon a pleasing appearance in other human beings and indeed in ourselves and the errors in those judgments in value.[13]

Clinicians must, in other words, never forget how difficult it is to be one of their patients, looked on as ugly and rejected by society. This insight should not come as a surprise, but it always does. Isaiah the prophet told us what our Savior would look like. Nonetheless, he always startles us when we meet him, "so marred [is] his appearance, beyond human semblance, and his form beyond that of mortals" (Is 52:14). Without understanding who it is that they are treating, clinicians will never have compassion and will never understand the limits of their craft. They need to see the beauty of Truth and Goodness that lie beneath appearances if they are ever to help their patients. In so doing, clinicians can come to understand who they are as moral agents and teach the rest of us hard lessons about life and its ultimate right values.

Hermanus Contractus

I would now like to illustrate the meaning of this approach to patient care by telling a story. The story is an old biography that was rediscovered and presented to the modern world by British Jesuit C. C. Martindale in the 1930s—the life of Hermann the Cripple. The abbreviated version I will recount here is an English translation of Father Luigi Giussani's very loose recounting of the story in Italian.[14]

On July 18, 1013, a son was born to Wolfrad, count of Althausen in Swabia, and his wife, Hiltrud. They came from very fine families. Noblemen, crusaders, and great prelates populated their pedigrees. Yet none of them do we remember, save the little fellow who was born most horribly deformed. He was so hideously distorted that afterward he was nicknamed "The Contracted." He could not stand, let alone walk. He could hardly sit, even in the special chair they made for him. Even his fingers were too weak and knotted for him to write. His mouth and palate were so deformed that he could barely be understood when he spoke.

In a pagan world he would, without argument, have been exposed at birth and left to perish. Modern pagans, especially when they observe that he was one of fifteen children, would announce that he never should have been born. Becoming still more logical, they would announce that he should have been painlessly put out of the way with an abortion. And they would say so all the more when I tell you that he appeared, to the judges of one thousand years ago, to be what we would today call a "defective." What did his parents, skulking about in the mud of those "Dark Ages" (as we have the nerve to call them), actually do? They sent him to a monastery, and they prayed.

It was the monasteries that had preserved and developed what they could from the ancient Roman and Greek civilizations. That culture came to Germany not only from the Latin south but also by way of visiting English and Irish monks. German translations of the Gospel were appearing; German sermons were being preached; hardly a great name in Latin or Greek failed to become known in this way. Most often, this scholarship and teaching occurred through the monasteries. Some of the great ones, such as St. Gall, Fulda, and Reichenau, established vast libraries.

To one such monastery, this little one, regarded as a defective freak, was sent. Reichenau was founded on a lovely little island situated in

Lake Constance just upstream from the beautiful falls of the River Rhine. This monastery had existed before Charlemagne—for some two hundred years before Hermann entered its gates. By the high road on the opposite shore, Italian, Greek, Irish, and even Icelandic travelers passed to and fro.

Reichenau sheltered famous scholars. It had its own school of painting—tenth-century paintings at St. Georg's Church in Oberzell and eleventh-century paintings at St. Peter's in Niederzell—all made by monks with the heart, if not yet the hand, of Fra Angelico. It was here in the monastery at Reichenau that the boy grew up. Here the lad who could hardly stammer with his tongue found his mind developing under something that we might today call "religious psychotherapy." Not once in his life would he have been comfortable or free of pain; yet what are the adjectives that were used to describe him? We read that he was "pleasant, friendly, easy to talk to, always laughing, never criticizing, eagerly cheerful." As a result, everybody loved him. And meanwhile the courageous lad—never, remember, at his ease in a chair nor so much as flat in bed—learned mathematics, Latin, Greek, Arabic, astronomy, and music. He wrote a whole treatise on the astrolabes, an instrument of navigation that preceded the sextant.

The preface of the original Latin text of this treatise on the astrolabes says: "Hermann, the least of the Christ's poor ones, and an amateur philosopher; a follower slower than any donkey, yes, slower than any snail, has been asked constantly by his friends to describe the system of the Astrolabes more fully and more clearly. . . . I had tried to wriggle out of doing so, making all sort of excuses, but really motivated by my lumpish laziness. At long last I have put my limp and hesitating hand to the work." Perhaps even more remarkable, with those twisted fingers the indomitable lad actually *made* astrolabes, and he also built clocks and musical instruments: never conquered, never idle!

And as for music—would that our modern choirs could read and sing his music! Hermann once wrote that a competent musician ought to be able to compose a reasonable tune, or anyway to judge it, and, finally, to sing it. "Most singers," he said, "attend to the third point only, and never think. They sing, or rather howl, not realizing that no one can sing properly if his thought is out of harmony with his voice. To such songsters loud voice is everything. This is worse than donkeys, which, after all, do make more noise, but never mix up braying with bellowing."

Hermann further observed that no one tolerates grammatical mistakes, yet the rules of grammar are artificial, whereas "music springs straight from nature," and therein not only do men fail to correct their faults, but they actually defend them. (You may detect a note of sarcasm. He could use, when he wanted to, a rather caustic tongue!) Yet it is thought that it was he who wrote the glorious hymn "Salve Regina," with its plain chant melody, which is still used today all over the Catholic world. He is also purported to have written the "Alma Redemptoris Mater" and many other hymns.

Moreover, Hermann, with his active and vigorous brain, wrote a chronicon, or world history from Christ's day to his own. Experts say that it was amazingly accurate—retelling tradition, of course, yet objective and original. Here, then, you have the crippled monk in his cell, alert, eyes wide open to the outside world, yet never cynical, never cruel (so many chronic sufferers grow cruel), making a complete perspective of the currents of life in Europe.

Well, the time at last came for him to die. His friend and historian Berthold described it this way: "When at the last the loving kindliness of God was deigning to free his holy soul from the tedious prison of this world, he was attacked by pleurisy, and for ten days spent almost all the time in agony. At last, one day, very early in the morning, after Mass, I, whom he counted his closest friend, went and asked him if he felt a little better. 'Do not ask me about that,' he answered, 'not about that! Listen carefully. I shall certainly die very soon. I shall not live. I shall not recover.'"

According to Berthold, Hermann went on to say how during the night he had felt as if he were rereading Cicero's *Hortensius*, with its wise sayings about right and wrong, and going over in his mind all that he himself had meant to write on the subject. And under the strong inspiration of this work, Hermann continued, "The whole of this present world and all that belongs to it, yes this mortal life itself has become mean and wearisome, and on the other hand, the world to come, that shall not pass, and the eternal life, have become so unspeakably desirable and dear, that I hold all these passing things as light as thistledown. I am tired of living."

When Hermann spoke thus, Berthold broke down completely, and in a fit of agitation cried, unable to control himself. After a while, Berthold related, Hermann "quite indignantly upbraided me, trembling and looking at me sideways with puzzled eyes."

"Heart's beloved," said Hermann, "do not weep, do not weep for me." And addressing one final message to Berthold, he added, "By remembering daily that you too are to die, prepare yourself with all your energy for the same journey, for, on some day and hour, you know not when, you shall follow me forth, me, your dear, dear friend." And, on these words, he expired.

Hermann died after receiving the Holy Communion on September 24, 1054, among all his friends, and he was buried—hidden little monk as he had been—amid great lamentations in his own estate of Althausen, which he had given up so long ago.

Hermann was a gift from God, radiant with Beauty, pining for Truth, awesome in his Goodness. Today we might have been able to correct some of his deformities. One cannot help but speculate whether his accomplishments would have been the same had his anomalies been corrected. But whether or not the deformities were correctable or treatable, Hermann could have been any of us. He gave much to his monastic community, to his country, and to his world, and he keeps on giving to us today through his story and through his music. He was not beautiful to behold, but he was beautiful in his Goodness. May we have the courage and the vision to count all the Hermanns we treat as among the greatest gifts God gives us.

CHAPTER 5

The Prodigal Profession

THE lofty vision I have sketched out in the first few chapters of this book may seem far from the reality of contemporary health care. Much has happened to the healing professions over the last fifty years. Unprecedented changes have swept through medicine, and these changes have affected physicians especially deeply. I see it when I compare the attitudes of my own medical school professors (particularly those who were already senior then) with those of my junior colleagues now. I sense it in what practitioners say and do now compared with my own experiences as a young boy visiting our family physician. Although many physicians are undoubtedly saints, as a whole, one could say that physicians today constitute a "prodigal profession." As a group, as a social institution, as a profession, physicians seem to have lost their way. In the depths of our hearts, we know this to be true. Those of us who practice this profession will never find our way back home unless we recognize how lost we have become.

The parable of the prodigal son is probably familiar. But because few have ever thought about what it might have to say about health care, it is worth recounting the story.

> There was a man who had two sons. The younger of them said to his father, "Father, give me the share of the property that will belong to me." So he divided his property between them. A few days later the younger son gathered all he had and traveled to a distant country, and there he squandered his property in dissolute living. When he had spent everything, a severe famine took place throughout that country, and he began to be in need. So he went and hired himself out to one of the citizens of that country, who sent him to his fields to feed the pigs. He

would gladly have filled himself with the pods that the pigs were eating; and no one gave him anything. But when he came to himself he said, "How many of my father's hired hands have bread enough and to spare, but here I am dying of hunger! I will get up and go to my father, and I will say to him, 'Father, I have sinned against heaven and before you; I am no longer worthy to be called your son; treat me like one of your hired hands.'" So he set off and went to his father. But while he was still far off, his father saw him and was filled with compassion; he ran and put his arms around him and kissed him. Then the son said to him, "Father, I have sinned against heaven and before you; I am no longer worthy to be called your son." But the father said to his slaves, "Quickly, bring out a robe—the best one—and put it on him; put a ring on his finger and sandals on his feet. And get the fatted calf and kill it, and let us eat and celebrate; for this son of mine was dead and is alive again; he was lost and is found!" And they began to celebrate. Now his elder son was in the field; and when he came and approached the house, he heard music and dancing. He called one of the slaves and asked what was going on. He replied, "Your brother has come, and your father has killed the fatted calf, because he has got him back safe and sound." Then he became angry and refused to go in. His father came out and began to plead with him. But he answered his father, "Listen! For all these years I have been working like a slave for you, and I have never disobeyed your command; yet you have never given me even a young goat so that I might celebrate with my friends. But when this son of yours came back, who has devoured your property with prostitutes, you killed the fatted calf for him!" Then the father said to him, "Son, you are always with me, and all that is mine is yours. But we had to celebrate and rejoice, because this brother of yours was dead and has come to life; he was lost and has been found." (Lk 15:11–24)

Spending Our Inheritance

Like the prodigal son, we physicians, as a profession, have squandered our common patrimony on dissolute living for several generations. In the last century and a half, we physicians have enjoyed untold successes. Medicine can now help and even cure diseases that the first twenty-three centuries of Western medical practitioners could not even imagine treatable. Modern health care can prevent infections with vaccines and prevent osteoporotic fractures with specific drugs. Physicians can prescribe hormones when patients cannot make their own. Antibiotics, so powerful and yet so commonplace, are only a bit more than sixty years old. Physicians now thread catheters into the coronary arteries of real human beings, inject dye, investigate, and even correct their anatomy. They open people's hearts, fix their valves and arteries, close them up, and not only do the patients survive but physicians now actually extend their lives and relieve their symptoms. Radiologists routinely put people inside huge magnets, bombard them with radio waves, and explore the inner workings of their brains. Oncologists give people drugs when their bodies are riddled with cancer, and the cancers go away. Some conditions, such as Hodgkin's disease and testicular cancer, are actually cured. Hippocrates could not have imagined this possible. We now consider it all routine.

Our scientific prowess has become immense. For example, just a few years ago, people in Lyme, Connecticut, began to suffer from a strange chronic arthritis. Physician-scientists conducted some epidemiological and microbiological research, developed an antibody test, performed a few clinical trials, and voilà—in a few short years, they had licked Lyme disease. Cures for cancer and AIDS are just around the corner. We are just a scan or two, a nucleotide or two, or a stem cell or two away.

Physicians have also learned to make quite a good living in this era of success. In some cases, if my fellow physicians and I are honest, it is too good a living. Certainly, no physician is starving.

So, things should be pretty good for physicians. We should be exceedingly happy. And so thought the prodigal son when he set off to spend his inheritance. And I am sure things *were* great, for a while. But eventually, one's transgressions always catch up. Dissolute living leads inevitably to dissolution. As a result, despite all the good news, despite the fact that we are capable of doing so much more for our patients than our predecessors could for theirs, health care professionals today are among the most dissatisfied of all professions in the United States.

Dissolute Living Leads to Dissolution

How is it that medicine's triumphs have brought such emptiness? What has gone awry?

First, it seems to me that we physicians have become too taken up with our own success. It has become quite easy for each of us to believe that we are in total command of all this technology; we are convinced that the power comes from us and belongs to us. We are hot stuff. People even pretend to play us on TV.

Many physicians put far too great a faith in the march of scientific progress in medicine. They have begun to harbor the belief that there is no health care problem that science cannot solve. If we just do enough research, use enough machines, or throw enough money at "it" (whatever "it" is), we can solve it.

Too many individual practitioners also believe too deeply in their own individual technological prowess. And why shouldn't they? They have seen it work. They seem to be saying, "Who needs to pray for miracles? We create our own." Physicians have become true believers.

And so have patients. This should also come as no surprise. Physicians have been telling the public for years how powerful and important they are. Now patients really believe them, so much so that physicians have become the great heroes of TV—Dr. Kildare, Marcus Welby, the staff of ER, and, currently, Dr. Gregory House, medical sleuth. No television news show is complete without having hyped some ever newer and greater medical breakthrough. Physicians have told patients that they are great. Patients have introjected the message, and now they play back the tape. On hearing it from their patients, physicians believe it all the more. This is operant conditioning at its best. B. F. Skinner would be very proud.

Physicians and patients are now both equally fascinated by the dials, the machines, the switches, the injections, and the pills. Physicians pull the levers and dispense the powerful drugs. Want to lose weight? Take a pill. Want to quit smoking? Take a pill. Want to feel happy? Take a pill. Stop going bald? Take a pill. Have children? Take a pill. Not have children? Take a pill. Live forever?

Patients want answers, and physicians write prescriptions.

Second, technology has begun to bite back. The burdens of illness inadvertently introduced by medical treatment grow daily. Most "buffalo humps" and "moon facies," types of abnormal fat deposits, are caused by physicians prescribing prednisone, not by pituitary tumors secreting hormones. The dreaded vancomycin-resistant enterococcus, a treatment-resistant bacterium, was concocted in the laboratory of physicians' own exuberant, frankly arrogant practices. The prodigal use of antibiotics has created the multiply-resistant "super germs" that now contaminate our intensive care units. Medical students and residents are still learning primarily in hospitals, which are increasingly becoming the places in which physicians manage the complications of treatment, such as chemotherapy-induced drops in blood count, the tearing of blood vessels after catheterization, or infections resulting from surgery.

More and more, patients feel imprisoned by the very technology that was supposed to set them free. The intensive care unit, the paradigmatic symbol of the technological prowess of medicine, the "Twilight Zone" where physicians "control the horizontal" and physicians "control the vertical," has become for many persons the symbol of the worst fate that could befall them. Patients feel increasingly alienated from their physicians, nurses, dentists, and other health care professionals. They feel depersonalized and dehumanized, as if they were extraordinarily complex biological machines at the mercy of mechanics and engineers.

Increasingly, health care professionals themselves are also becoming alienated from their work. Once their labors come to be viewed as mere expertise and technology, looking through a scope and inspecting human colons a dozen times a day can become as boring as inspecting chickens in a poultry-processing plant. Both are just applied science—the practical use of highly specialized knowledge.

Third, the financing of health care is shifting dramatically and rapidly. Under the old fee-for-service system, too many physicians behaved as what I have called "factitious" gatekeepers—creating the illusion of consumer demand for services that were not really medically necessary, lining their pockets in the process. Very few have done this consciously, of course. But quite a few members of the profession have done so at least unconsciously. The evidence is overwhelming. For example, if a physician owns a share in a free-standing MRI facility, his or her patients are more likely to get MRIs.[1]

And collectively, throughout this century, medical professional organizations have functioned very much like trade unions. They have united to fight against every genuine attempt at health care reform.[2] And when they could not stop partial attempts at reform (such as Medicare), they found ways to make it work for their own self-interest. Organized professional medicine has consistently worked against the care of the poor in this country in order to protect professional income, with great success.

Physicians now stand accused of having spent other people's money wantonly for decades. And this has become the justification for turning physicians into depersonalized cogs in the wheel of corporate medicine. Managed care is an attempt to use industrial techniques to control the inflation-generating technological exuberance of physicians and their patients. Efficiency has become physicians' most cherished virtue. How many "resource utilizing units" (i.e., patients) did that "provider" (i.e., doctor) service at what "medical loss ratio" with respect to potential shareholder profit?

Physicians have become used to complaining about all this, and justifiably so. People blame them for taking up 15 percent of the gross national product. Now, that 15 percent of the economy is in utter financial chaos.

Why Did We Leave Our Father's Mansion?

What has become of the human person in the midst of all this? The question is too rarely asked.

Too often, the patient has become merely the context in which physicians display their power. What they find important is their power, not the good of the patient. All talk to the contrary is now dismissed as silly, anachronistic, idealistic tomfoolery. Patients are consumers—amorphous blobs of undifferentiated medical preferences. Physicians are the providers. They provide the power—the means of satisfying consumer demand. There is nothing very personal to all this. It is about supply and demand for gadgets and pills.

New time pressures have resulted in complex changes in physician behavior. In order to maintain income when the amount paid per visit has been ratcheted down by third-party payers, physicians have decreased the time they spend with each patient in order to increase volume and see more patients per day in the office. Internists (at least those who have not yet been replaced by hospitalists and therefore still visit their own patients in the hospital) now often perform hospital rounds at 6 A.M.—to avoid wasting time by encountering families.

Physicians find themselves caught in a system of health care financing that presumes that patients and physicians are greedy, essentially self-interested, and incapable of altruism. This system proposes to harness physician self-interest in order to control costs and make more money for the entrepreneurs. Yet, paradoxically, physicians are told that their professional integrity must remain in place as the sole means of protecting patients against exploitation in the present system. No wonder so many physicians feel confused!

Physicians also sometimes find themselves caught in a web of lies reminiscent of a Solzhenitsyn novel. Physicians regularly supply "doctored" information on behalf of their patients in order to secure reasonable care from insurance companies.[3] Although it is morally wrong, it is easy to see how this happens.

For instance, it is well established that the most common illnesses treated by internists are psychological—depression, anxiety, and somatization ("psychosomatic illness"). In the mid-1990s, however, managed care organizations began to implement policies that would not pay for psychiatric care by general internists or family physicians, arguing that these physicians were not qualified to care for these disorders. Most general internists and family physicians are, in fact, clearly capable of treating these disorders with antidepressants or antianxiety drugs. Nonetheless, seeing psychiatrists, true specialists in these disorders, is sometimes better for some of these patients. Furthermore, patients with somatization disorder will almost never admit that the root cause of their symptoms is psychological. They rarely present dangers to themselves, but they fiercely resist seeing psychiatrists and return over and over again to internists and family physicians. Still, the managed care organizations not only began to refuse to pay for the care that internists and family physicians provided for these conditions but also often had contractual clauses in patients' policies that required that these patients be suicidal in order to be approved to see psychiatrists. This created a classic catch-22 situation for patients who suffered from quite severe (and quite treatable) psychiatric illnesses. According to the insurance company's rules, they were too complexly ill to warrant treatment by generalists and not sick enough to be seen by the specialists.

As a general internist working in a university medical center's faculty practice in the mid-1990s, I was told by our business managers that the faculty practice could be reimbursed only for treating organic illnesses or symptoms, not psychiatric disorders. So I was told to fill out billing slips that reported symptoms but not the actual diagnoses for patients who were psychiatrically ill. Compounding the matter, there were only a limited number of symptoms that one could check off from the list on our standard billing form. If we were to write in a symptom not listed on the billing form, the chances were that the delay necessary in order to have the symptom-related code entered by a clerk would result in a denial of payment due to late submission of the charges. And the already depressed patient would then receive a personal bill demanding cash payment, saying that our services had not been covered by their policy. Thus, if I saw a depressed patient who had difficulty concentrating, the inability to feel pleasure, loss of appetite, depressed mood, early morning awakening, and suicidal thoughts but without any committed suicidal intention or plan, I went ahead and treated the patient. But I was informed that I should write "sleep disturbance" on our billing forms rather than "depression" in order to be reimbursed. Everyone knew this was substantially less than the whole truth. But everyone was expected to do it. Even the insurance company knew it was being done. The system had become completely dependent on lying in order to function. After numerous complaints and lawsuits from practitioners and patients, this situation has largely disappeared. But similar new bureaucratic nightmares are emerging all the time.

All told, then, it is easy to understand why so many physicians are becoming cynical and bitter. Physicians have been knocked off their pedestals. Their expertise has been popularly reinterpreted as thinly disguised greed. Now, physicians are regarded as heroes *only* on television. In real life, physicians are greeted everywhere with suspicion. Whenever anything goes wrong, physicians are quick to blame patients, and patients are quick to blame their physicians. But for physicians, there is one very big rub—disgruntled patients bring lawsuits.

Responsibility and Repentance

There are plenty of causes for the current situation. Many are due to social and economic forces that are much broader than health care. All I want to suggest is that physicians cannot blame every bit of this on others. We set out decades ago on a prodigal path, and now that the famine is upon us, we do not have the wherewithal to survive it on our own. We physicians must be honest enough to note that we are partially responsible for creating this crisis. We physicians must share the blame for what has happened to us. The frustrations of many have reached a point of near desperation. And our crisis is primarily spiritual. We are dying of spiritual starvation.

The prodigal son, after all, is not depicted in the parable as horrible, vicious, and vile. The prodigal son was just a bit reckless, just a bit haughty, just a bit arrogant. The prodigal son simply forgot some basic truths, and basic relationships, and set out to live by his own lights, alone. And he got lost.

Many physicians today are in a state similar to that of the prodigal son. They are lost, buried in mounds of paper. They are hurt, because their patients no longer trust them. They are dissatisfied, because their practices have become so depersonalized. They are bewildered, wondering how it all could have happened. Like the prodigal son they suddenly find themselves, once proud, independent, and vain, now attached to the "propertied class"—the entrepreneurs and the MBAs. They are now led around by the nose by people whose greed far exceeds any of which physicians have ever been accused. And yet the blame meted out by patients still falls on the physicians. Clinging to some semblance of their former moral codes, physicians now find themselves daily facing moral stress tests under the new payment structures— asking themselves how much they are willing to compromise their own financial interests in order to help their patients.

Those of us who are physicians know in our hearts that there is a better way. We are starving for that way. Our clinical hunger for rendering compassionate care persists. But we are caught in a world of alienation, deceit, greed, and technocratic indifference—a deep spiritual famine. Like the prodigal son, the prodigal profession finds itself scrounging for scraps of meaning in a system of health care that is increasingly devoid of meaning. The gnawing feeling in our bellies when we return from work each night, in frustration with the system and with ourselves, is not caused by *Helicobacter pylori* (the bacteria that causes ulcers). The only source of satisfaction for our spiritual hunger is God.

Una Selva Oscura

Dante's *Divine Comedy* begins this way—

> Nel mezzo del cammin di nostra vita
> Mi ritrovai in una selva oscura.

[In the middle of the course of our life,
I found myself in a dark wood.][4]

As sons and daughters of Adam and of Hippocrates, as brothers and sisters in Christ, this is where we physicians find ourselves today: in the middle of a dark wood, lost, prodigal, dissolute in spirit. We physicians have only one important question to ask ourselves, like the question the prodigal son asked himself. Each must ask, "When will I come to my senses and return to my Father?"

To ask this, physicians need first to realize how lost they have become. They must recognize, contritely, their own role in losing their way. As a collectivity, as a profession, physicians today have largely squandered the inheritance of Hippocrates, of Cosmos and Damien, of Christ the Great Physician, from whom they have received every good gift of healing. When will they come to their senses, ask forgiveness, and return to their Father?

The medical profession cannot, and will not, be reformed as a profession unless and until each physician has been reformed in his or her own heart. The prodigal profession will not return to its roots because of a resolution by the American Medical Association. I suggest four ways in which physicians can begin the change of heart that Gospel healing demands of them, four ways in which they can begin to discover anew the spiritual meaning that has always been at the heart of health care, four ways that the prodigal profession can begin the journey back to its spiritual home.

1. *Physicians can begin to recover the sense that the encounter with the patient is an encounter with the holy mystery of God.* The work with which physicians are engaged is not a mere exchange of goods and services, but the stuff of religious experience, if only they can awaken themselves to the awesome mysteries that unfold before them. They come into the presence of God countless times each day. God comes to physicians naked, cold, outcast, suffering, and sick. Physicians may ask, "Lord, when did we see you sick and comfort you?" And the Lord answers, "Whenever you did something for the least of my brothers and sisters, you did it for me."

We physicians need to rekindle this spirit. We need to learn once again to treat our patients with reverent attentiveness. We need to find ways to remind ourselves that God has freely chosen to come to us, humbly, through their sufferings and that God is also present as the grace that motivates our offer to help. I know one physician, for instance, who stops and stands still for ten seconds before seeing each patient—just ten simple silent seconds of stillness—in order to recollect himself before entering the exam room of each patient. Others pray for their patients at night, recalling who they saw that day, individually and prayerfully recollecting them, and commending them and their needs to God. In the end, the method does not matter much. What matters is that each physician should find a way to hear the call to come home. If we hear that call, I have faith that we each can find our own way back.

2. *Physicians would do well to recall that the relationship between health care professionals and patients demands trust.* Patients are exceedingly vulnerable and often desperate. They do not have the means of discovering what is wrong with them or what can be done about it. That is why they come to physicians. Physicians have the knowledge and the power. Patients are forced to trust in their physicians. Let us pray that those of us who are physicians will live professional lives worthy of our patients' trust.

I once spoke with a friend who wanted advice about an orthopedic surgeon. His first shoulder surgery to repair a torn rotator cuff had not resulted in a very good outcome. What annoyed him most was not that the outcome had been bad but that the surgeon had ignored all his complaints postoperatively until a year later, when an MRI revealed the problem. My friend then called me for advice. He wanted my guidance in helping him to choose another surgeon. He was really agonizing over the choice. He wanted someone whom he could trust would be competent, compassionate, and honest. He knew he ultimately had to trust someone—that he would need to trust someone to put him to sleep, stick his fingers in his shoulder, make cuts, sew tendons, close him up, and stay there with him through months of recovery. I ended our telephone conversation by assuring him that I would pray that the person he would eventually choose would be worthy of that trust.

3. *Physicians would do well to remember that the power to heal does not belong to them but to God.* Physicians can only predispose their patients to healing. In the end, it is God who heals. It would be a great blessing

for patients if physicians were always humble enough to remember that and to be grateful to God for the awesome mystery of healing.

No individual practitioner, living or deceased, invented medicine or dentistry or nursing from scratch. First, all the knowledge that practitioners have has been given to them through their teachers. They should be grateful to God for their teachers. Second, as the Book of Sirach (38:1–8) so strongly points out, their teachers' teachers' teachers learned the art from observing the healing gifts of the world God has created. Physicians and all health care practitioners should be grateful to God for the healing powers in nature. Third, the ability to learn all this information came to them as a free gift from God. Physicians, nurses, dentists, and psychologists did not give themselves the intelligence and ability to learn the healing arts. They should be grateful to God for the talents he has given each of them. Finally, every medical act depends on the body's own regenerative powers. The surgeon cuts, and he predisposes the body to healing. But it is the patient's own body that recovers from the surgery. If wounds did not heal independent of the surgeon, there could be no surgery. Similarly, antibiotics do not cure without an immune system. Diuretics do not help congestive heart failure without a kidney. Physicians simply never heal independent of God, and it is only immense vanity that would make them think differently.

In the words of Ben Sira (38:2, 4–8), "Their gift of healing comes from the Most High. . . . The Lord created medicines out of the earth, and the sensible will not despise them. And he gave skill to human beings that he might be glorified in his marvelous works. By them the physician heals and takes away pain; the pharmacist makes a mixture from them. God's works will never be finished; and from him health spreads over all the earth."

Physicians might cultivate a deeper sense of wonder at medical science. Now that the human genome project has been completed, and every last nucleotide is known, how could anyone think that we thereby have figured out the mystery of the human? That mystery is the axis around which the double helix is coiled. It cannot be seen or touched, but without it there is no human being. How fearfully, wonderfully are we made (Ps 139:14). How privileged are those of us in the health care professions who learn such wonders in such depth. Let us praise God for those wonders, not lose sight of the mysteries of the embodied human person. And let us never be so arrogant as to claim that we own or control these mysteries. "Not to us, O Lord, not to us, but to Your name give glory" (Ps 115:1).

4. *Physicians can make a renewed commitment to health care as service.* They can learn to see their scientific knowledge as an opportunity for service, not for control. They can learn again to live the Liturgy of the Lord's Supper, commemorating in deed as well as in symbol the example Christ offers in the washing of feet. This is the model of discipleship. Those who claim to know Jesus and to follow him must imitate his example of service.

Jesus does not command that a spirit of service should be cultivated because it makes good business sense. A true disciple of Christ does not set out to make the patients feel welcome so that they will purchase more health care services. The Gospel is not a marketing ploy. The Gospel teaches us to serve our patients for the sake of serving them. The Gospel calls us to love our patients. We show our love for them by recognizing each and every one of them as created in the image and likeness of God, endowed with an indelible dignity, serving them with reverent attention because we recognize the divine spark within each of them. Patients should count in our eyes because they count in God's eyes—young and old; rich and poor; black, white, Latino, and Asian; the athletes and the paralyzed; the brilliant and the retarded. Let us wash their feet.

Spirit and Truth

Physicians cannot change all the social forces that have recently beset their noble profession. But they can, by cooperating with God's grace, change themselves. They can refuse to sell their Hippocratic souls. They can persevere in prayer and in caring attitudes. They can remember that the social, political, and economic environment does not change the fundamental human realities of sickness, death, and healing. They can maintain faith and hope.

Concluding Prayer

So bring us back, O Lord. I pray to you, bring us back home. We, your prodigal sons and daughters, have wandered far from you. We have lived dissolute professional lives, and we now feel the inevitable dissolution. Convert our hearts. As we starve for spiritual food, help us to recall the bounty of your table.

Teach us to see again—that in the wounds of our patients we may see your wounds—the wounds by which all of us are healed.

Teach us to hear again—that when we place our stethoscopes on the chests of our patients we may hear the plaintive beating of your own Most Sacred Heart.

Teach us to feel again—that our own coldness may vanish as we touch the fevered skin of the sick; that like you, when people reach out to us asking for healing, we may recognize the divine power of healing that goes out from us.

Let us look to that day of great rejoicing, when patients and healers can go home together to the house of their one Father to celebrate the triumph of life; to cheer as the prodigal profession, once lost, discovers itself again and is finally found.

CHAPTER 6

Aesculapion

*I*T is hard to trust a profession that cannot even get its symbols straight. Most physicians in the United States think that the symbol of their healing profession is something called the caduceus. But this is actually not true.

A caduceus is a gold or polished bronze rod with a pair of wings at the top and two snakes twisted about it. I am sure it is familiar to most persons. It is depicted on the seals of several U.S. medical schools. Medical students and undergraduate premed students at several schools belong to clubs named the Caduceus Club. Student newspapers at several medical schools are called the *Caduceus* and use this symbol on their mastheads. Microsoft Word's clip art package uses the caduceus as its "health care and medicine" symbol. It may be ubiquitous, but this symbol has nothing to do with the ancient traditions of Greek and Roman medicine. The caduceus is actually the symbol of Hermes or Mercury, the winged messenger god.

The true symbol of medicine is the Aesculapion, the symbol of Aesculapius, the hero-physician of ancient Greek mythology from whom Hippocrates claimed descent. The Aesculapion is similar to the caduceus but differs in important ways. The Aesculapion is a rather gnarled, wingless, wooden staff with a single snake wrapped about it. Historians have discovered that someone in the U.S. Army Medical Corps mistook the caduceus for the Aesculapion and introduced the caduceus as the Medical Corps' symbol at the beginning of the twentieth century. Soon thereafter, everyone in the United States was emulating the mistake.[1]

Snake Stories

It turns out that the myth of the Aesculapion is interesting, particularly for health professionals who are Jewish or Christian. In the Exodus story, Moses cures the Israelites who have been bitten by saraph serpents when, at God's command, he fashions a serpent made from bronze and holds it before the victims so that they may gaze on it (Nm 21:4–9). In the Gospel of John, Christ makes an allusion to this Exodus story, imbuing it with prophetic meaning in light of his Passion. "Just as Moses lifted up the serpent in the desert, so must the Son of Man be lifted up" (Jn 3:14).

As the ancient Romans and Greeks tell it, Aesculapius, the mythical hero-healer, was called one day to attend to a man named Glaucus, who had been struck by lightning. While he was attending to the patient, a snake slithered into the room. Distracted from his work, Aesculapius struck the snake with his wooden staff and killed it. Soon, a second snake arrived, carrying herbs in its mouth. As Aesculapius watched in amazement, the second snake used its tongue to place the herbs in the mouth of the dead snake, whereupon the dead snake came back to life. Aesculapius got the message. He took some of the herbs and placed them in the mouth of Glaucus, who was immediately revived. Subsequently, Aesculapius fashioned a symbol for himself—a snake wrapped around a wooden staff. This symbol, the Aesculapion, became the symbol of the medical profession.[2]

The story of Moses and the saraph serpent appears to be older than the Greek myth. Whether the Greeks borrowed the story from the Jews or came on it independently does not matter. All people of good will have at least some access to God's truth, even if it is not what Christians hold as the fullness of God's truth. The anthropological truth is that healing is associated symbolically with a snake. The deeper level of meaning, for believing Christians, is that Jesus says in the scriptures that this snake is a symbol for him. What such a claim might mean will require more than superficial reflection.

Although in some ancient cultures serpents were considered symbols of fertility and life, they are more commonly considered symbols of evil. The suggestive ambiguity between these two symbolic meanings notwithstanding, the latter seems to be more common in the scriptures. The tempter in the Garden of Eden is a serpent (Gn 3). In the Book of Revelation, the woman clothed with the sun is locked in mortal struggle with the serpent, explicitly described as a symbol of Satan (Rv 12). The saraph serpents in the story from the Book of Numbers are a punishment (Nm 21:4–9). They are sent by God to bite the Israelites in retribution for their grumbling.

Snakes evoke deep fears in people. Some are lethally poisonous. Many people have snake phobias. These reptiles appear in dreams as signs of our subconscious fears. How could such a symbol evoke healing? How could a snake be a symbol for Christ?

Formal exegesis aside, one way to start thinking about such questions is by searching for the serpents in one's own life. "Serpents" abound. One probably need not look very far.

The Book of Numbers (21:4–5) explains why the saraph serpents appeared in the desert, and the meaning of these words traverses the centuries: "But the people became impatient on the way. The people spoke against God and Moses." The following litany evokes the doctor's dining room, does it not?

> "HMOs. PPOs. DRGs. OMB. IRS. CLIA. HIPAA."
> "Snakes. All of them—snakes."
> "Why did I enter this wretched profession anyway? Things were so much better in the past. I can see no promised land ahead."

Many physicians today feel as if they are wandering in a desert—they have left behind the land of the pharaoh, but they are uncertain where the journey will end. And many of the things they have created are now biting back.[3] This is a sad truth about all technology, but it is especially true of medical technology. As I discussed in the last chapter, the medical profession has practically promised immortality to patients. Is it any wonder that patients now sue physicians so readily when things go wrong? The overexuberant use of antibiotics to treat one set of infections has created new infectious diseases, such as C. dificile colitis and methicillin-resistant staph aureus. Technology now helps people to live longer, but this very success may mean that they live long enough to develop degenerative disorders, such as Alzheimer disease. Things bite back. The truth is that if one worships technology as one's golden calf, the saraph serpents will follow.

And what about those dark serpents lurking inside those of us who practice the healing professions? If we are honest, many of us will recognize our own tendencies to actually resent patients as impositions on us, our tendencies to use patients to display our power, and those all-too-subtle tendencies to allow patient need to bleed over into our own self-interest. "I think everyone needs an annual EKG. Wouldn't want to miss anything." "Well, it's always better to be safe. Let's biopsy that mole."

And although there are some new serpents preying on our patients these days, most of the serpents that slither down the corridors of our hospitals are as old as sin and death. Among them are the brute facts of illness, injury, and mortality; the biting reality of pain; and the poisons of kidney disease, diabetes, and bacterial toxins. Patients now also suffer all too frequently from the poisons health care professionals give them in the name of therapy—immunological treatments such as inter-leukin-2, chemotherapeutic agents such as cis-platinum, anti-HIV drugs such as indinivir, and others. And patients, once bitten, can find themselves suffering from the most poisonous venom that can ever course through human veins—the venom of despair.

There is obviously no shortage of serpents in the world of health care. Facing so many, a rational person is bound to ask, who can save us from all this? Health care today seems adrift, wandering aimlessly, surrounded by venomous vipers. Surely (at least in our moments of sobriety) we realize that we cannot save ourselves.

A Saraph Savior?

But perhaps there is a remedy for the soul sickness that so many physicians, nurses, dentists, psychologists, and other health care professionals feel today. Perhaps there is a route through the desert. Perhaps there is a destination after all—a promised land. If so, it will not come from the House of Representatives or the National Institutes of Health or the Institute of Medicine. "For God so loved the world that he gave his only Son, so that he who believes in him may not perish but may have eternal life. Indeed God did not send the Son into the world to condemn the world, but that the world might be saved through him" (Jn 3:16–17).

We have a Savior—a saraph Savior. He is the One, the Good, the Holy Savior. He is the True Physician, the Source of all healing.

He takes up our pride
Our greed
Our resentment
Our pettiness;
He takes on our pain
Our suffering
Our nausea
Our fatigue
Our dyspnea
Our despair;
And he says, "Look at me."

In the second letter to the Corinthians, St. Paul writes, "For our sake he made him to be sin who did not know sin, so that, in him, we might become the righteousness of God" (2 Cor 5:21). This passage is often considered perplexing. What meaning does it portend for health care?

I think it means that all the sin and pain and sorrow of every patient and every practitioner—doctors, nurses, dentists, psychologists, chaplains—have been lifted up, wrapped around a pole, and nailed to a tree. I think both Moses and Jesus meant it when they said that to be saved, one must dare to look at the serpent.

So, these passages from the Book of Numbers and the Gospel of John turn out to have very practical implications for health care practitioners. The message seems to be that the Gospel way is not business as usual. Business as usual means running away from the serpents. Business as usual means hiding from one's own sinfulness. Business as usual means avoiding the deformed, the contagious, the retarded, the demented, the dying, and the needy.

But the truth that the Gospel proclaims is that try as one might to run away, there is no escape. Medicine is all about snakes, and they are everywhere. One cannot run away. There is no place to hide. If we were to try, the saraph serpents would just bite at our heels. What we fear comes back to get us.

The truth that the Gospel proclaims is that it is only by looking at the serpent that we can be saved—it is only by confronting our own sickness and sin (and that of others) that we can overcome sickness and sin. The Gospel makes some paradoxical demands: Go into the pain. Go into the sadness. Go into the fear. Go into the vipers' den.

This is what God did for us in Jesus—who humbled himself to take the form of a slave and remained obedient, even unto death.

One might justifiably inquire, however, what it could possibly mean to say that health care professionals usually run away from this serpent. It would seem that they face him every day. Not just anyone has the constitution to face the blood and pus that physicians and nurses face. In this way, of course, it is true that they do face the serpent—sin and sickness are everywhere in medicine. Yet, ironically, many physicians, nurses, psychologists, and other health care professionals try to deny or escape from this central reality of their profession.

Some ways of trying to avoid the snake are more obvious than others. For example, more physicians are now retiring early. But less obviously, some develop a posture of callous indifference toward the suffering of their patients, their families, themselves. Some pervert their professional calling into an entrepreneurial affair in which making money is what counts. It is easier to ignore the suffering of others if one can pretend that health care is a commodity. Others become cynical—a state that is not just pessimistic about the human predicament but actually takes perverse pleasure in being among the "enlightened" who know that all is folly.

But these are unhealthy states for practitioners, and they are deeply un-Christian attitudes. The Christian way of confronting the serpent cannot be with indifference or cynicism. Nor can it consist of an angry, hostile, indignant confrontation with the realities of suffering and sin. There is no escape from suffering. It bites us all. And health care professionals ought to know this better than anyone else.

Gazelles

A Saudi Arabian folktale can help to illustrate the above point.

> A Bedouin set out one day with his young son to take his camel grazing and to look for wild herbs and roots to take back for his wife to cook. When they had loaded up the camel and were heading home, a herd of magnificent gazelles suddenly appeared across their path. Silently and quickly the father made the camel lower herself to her knees. He slid from her back, and warning the boy not to stray, he hurried after the gazelles. The wild things leaped into the air and streaked off as soon as

he stepped toward them, but the Bedouin was a keen hunter. He eagerly followed their trail.

Meanwhile the young child waited alone. After all, there is no escape from destiny. As fate would have it, a She-Ghoul, that monster of the wilderness who loves to feed on human flesh, came upon the boy as he stood unprotected. With one leap she sprang upon him and greedily devoured him.

The father hunted long and far but could not catch a single gazelle. At last he resigned himself and returned without the game. Though the camel was kneeling where he had left it, he could not see his son. He looked around him on every side, but could not find the boy. Then on the ground he found dark drops of blood. "My son! My son is killed! My son is dead!" he shrieked. There was nothing more he could do but to lead his camel home.

On the way, he rode past a cave where he saw the She-Ghoul dancing, fresh from her feast, her hanging breasts swinging from side to side like the empty sleeves of women's cloaks when they rock in mourning over the dead. The Bedouin took careful aim and with one arrow shot the She-Ghoul dead. He slashed open her belly, and in it he found his son. He laid the boy upon his cloak, pulled the woolen cloth around him tight, and so carried him home.

When he reached his tent, he called his wife and said, "I have brought you back a gazelle, dear wife, but as God is my witness, it can be cooked only in a cauldron that has never been used for a meal of sorrow."

At her husband's request, the woman went from tent to tent, asking for the loan of such a pot. But one neighbor said, "Sister, we used our large cauldron to cook rice for the people who came to weep with us when my husband died." And another told her, "We last heated our big cooking pot on the day of my son's funeral." She knocked at every door but did not find what she sought. So she returned to her husband empty-handed.

"Haven't you found the right kind of cauldron?" asked the Bedouin.

"There is no household but has seen misfortune," she answered. "There is no cauldron but has cooked a meal of mourning."

Only then did the Bedouin fold back his woolen cloak and say to her, "They have all tasted their share of sorrow. Today is our turn. This is my gazelle."[4]

Although now rarely used in this way, the verb phrase "to suffer," in its most basic sense, means to undergo or to be the object of an action, regardless of whether it is pleasant or unpleasant, as in "to suffer a change." Equally important, the word "patient" is related, coming from the Latin *patiens*, for "one who suffers." In this most basic sense, *patient* is the opposite of agent—that which receives the action of a transitive verb as opposed to that which performs the action. Thus, suffering and being a patient are intimately linked linguistically. But beyond etymology, they share a common meaning. The most fundamental aspect of suffering is the fact that what one suffers is beyond one's control—suffering is what one undergoes, what happens, what one endures. One cannot control true suffering. Suffering is what remains when one's control runs out. And the very fact that it is beyond one's control means that it helps to define one's limits. To be a patient is to be one who suffers, and to suffer is to experience one's limits.

To understand suffering this way not only resonates deeply with the word's etymology. It may be precisely the understanding that the twenty-first century needs. More formally, I have argued that what it means for a human being to suffer is that the individual undergoes an experience that makes explicit the essential tension between the intrinsic dignity and the finitude that characterize human beings as a natural kind.[5] Although the pain of arthritis hurts, it is the fact that the pain prevents one from opening a jar that grounds the experience as an experience of suffering.

We experience ourselves and our fellow human beings as endowed with an incomparable worth or value—one that points us toward the infinite. This is our intrinsic dignity. But we also experience ourselves as limited—morally, intellectually, and biologically. We sin. We make mistakes. We become ill and die. This is our finitude. Dignity and finitude are both true of us as the kinds of things that we are, part of our essence. And dignity and finitude are in tension, for although we are necessarily finite, we are also oriented toward the infinite—to Goodness, to Truth, to Beauty, and to Life. Our status, compared with all other creatures in the known universe, makes us exalted. We are the sorts of creatures that are capable of moral agency, reason, aesthetic experience, worship, imagination, and more. But we fall short on all these counts. We wither like the grass. "Suffering" is the label we use to describe those experiences that make explicit the tension between these essential truths of our nature—that we are possessed of that great value we call dignity, yet we are finite creatures that are imperfect in body, mind, and soul.

In the Western world in the twenty-first century, people seem to think that limits are intrinsically evil. But this cannot be so. Limits define things. Without limits, there would be nothing but amorphous undifferentiated stuff. As Bishop Butler once remarked, "Everything is what it is, and not another thing."[6] All definitions must necessarily exclude some things and include other things. And so suffering, when we experience our limits in the face of our dignity, also serves to define us, helps us to understand who and what we are.[7]

This is what happens when we gaze on the serpent wrapped around the pole—we learn who and what we are. The wooden staff, upright and dignified, points to the infinite, while the serpent, the creature that is limited to crawling on the ground, points to the finite. It is in this space, poised between heaven and earth, at this point of intersection of the timeless with time, that we become human.

Really understanding this should heal us—heal us of our delusions of grandeur, heal us of our false beliefs that we can escape from suffering, heal us of the pervasive lie that we are superior to other human beings and capable of such escape. If we were thus fully healed, we would be compelled to acts of charity, full of the knowledge that anyone's suffering could have been ours. The suffering of our patients and our own suffering are thus subsumed under this symbol, pointing inexorably to the mystery of the human.

So the Christian way is to go face forward into the unavoidable pain of life—whether our own or that of our patients. The Christian way is to wrap one's dead son in a white cloth and carry him home in silence—like Mary leaving Golgotha. The Christian way is to gaze on the serpent and thereby understand the meaning of the prophesy, "They shall look on the one whom they have pierced" (Jn 19:37). There is no resurrection without crucifixion, no way to eternal life except through death.

And so a Christian meets the sickness and sin of the world

> With the charity of Christ;
> With the service of Christ;
> With the forgiveness of Christ.

This way is made possible for us only in the Spirit who is given to us. This means that Christian health care must be different—concretely—in the hospital and in the office. The Gospel must make a difference when the patient keeps complaining about her osteoarthritis because the anti-inflammatory drugs are not doing enough, and there are too many joints hurting to replace them all, and both you and the patient are frustrated. It must make a difference when the patient is dying, and you know that a mistake of yours was at least partly to blame. It must make a difference when an insurance clerk is telling you over the phone that the operation you plan to perform is not medically indicated. It must make a difference when your colleague is trying to persuade you to join him in accepting capitation fees from drug companies for enrolling patients in clinical trials.

Christ says: Do not run away. Do not be angry. Do not be cynical. Do not be afraid.

Embrace the leper. Embrace the prostitute with HIV. Embrace your burned-out colleague. And do not grumble about your lot. Meet the serpents of sickness and sin head on—

With the charity of Christ;
With the patience of Christ;
With the healing power of Christ.
After all, HE is the true symbol of our profession,
Who comes into your world not to condemn you or your patients,
But to save you.
For you know that you cannot save yourself.
All that you can do is to suffer the salvation that he offers you,
The Aesculapion—
The saraph mounted on the pole.
Everyone who believes in him will be healed.

CHAPTER 7

The Man Born Blind

ICONFESS that the Gospel of John frequently baffles me. I often find the writing terribly abstract: "I am in him and he is in me as I am in you and you are in me." It can sound at times like the lyrics from a Beatles' song, and I find myself wondering whether I would understand the secret message of John's Gospel any better if I were to find an old turntable to play it backward at 78 rpm. The Church is very big, however, and I am convinced that God authorized four Gospels in order that at least one would "work" for everyone. Given a choice of one of the four, I guess I would describe myself as kind of a "Luke guy," which is only to be expected of a narrow-minded physician. Luke, after all, *was* a physician.

Nonetheless, there are a few passages in the Gospel of John that I find very intimate, personal, and powerfully moving. These are John's descriptions of several intense encounters that Jesus had with individual persons. Jesus's conversation with the Samaritan woman at the well is one of these stories (Jn 4:4–42). The story of the man born blind from birth (Jn 9:1–41) is another. It is a story of drama and power, with much to tell health care professionals.

> As he walked along, he saw a man blind from birth. His disciples asked him, "Rabbi, who sinned, this man or his parents, that he was born blind?" Jesus answered, "Neither this man nor his parents sinned; he was born blind so that God's works might be revealed in him. We must work the works of him who sent me while it is day; night is coming when no one can work. As long as I am in the world, I am the light of the world." When he had said this, he spat on the ground and made mud with the saliva and spread the mud on the man's eyes, saying to him, "Go, wash

in the pool of Siloam" (which means Sent). Then he went and washed and came back able to see. The neighbors and those who had seen him before as a beggar began to ask, "Is this not the man who used to sit and beg?" Some were saying, "It is he." Others were saying, "No but it is someone like him." He kept saying, "I am the man." But they kept asking him, "Then how were your eyes opened?" He answered, "The man called Jesus made mud, spread it on my eyes, and said to me, 'Go to Siloam and wash.' Then I went and washed and received my sight." They said to him, "Where is he?" He said, "I do not know."

They brought to the Pharisees the man who had formerly been blind. Now it was a sabbath day when Jesus made the mud and opened his eyes. Then the Pharisees also began to ask him how he had received his sight. He said to them, "He put mud on my eyes. Then I washed, and now I see." Some of the Pharisees said, "This man is not from God, for he does not observe the sabbath." But others said, "How can a man who is a sinner perform such signs?" And they were divided. So they said again to the blind man, "What do you say about him? It was your eyes he opened." He said, "He is a prophet."

The Jews did not believe that he had been blind and had received his sight until they called the parents of the man who had received his sight and asked them, "Is this your son, who you say was born blind? How then does he now see?" His parents answered, "We know that this is our son, and that he was born blind; but we do not know how it is that now he sees, nor do we know who opened his eyes. Ask him; he is of age. He will speak for himself." His parents said this because they were afraid of the Jews; for the Jews had already agreed that anyone who confessed Jesus to be the Messiah would be put out of the synagogue. Therefore his parents said, "He is of age; ask him."

So for the second time they called the man who had been blind, and they said to him, "Give glory to God! We know that this man is a sinner." He answered, "I do not know whether he is a sinner. One thing I do know, that though I was blind, now I see." They said to him, "What did he do to you? How did he open your eyes?" He answered them, "I have told you already, and you would not listen. Why do you want to hear it again? Do you also want to become his disciples?" Then they reviled him, saying, "You are his disciple, but we are disciples of Moses. We know that God has spoken to Moses, but as for this man, we do not know where he comes from." The man answered, "Here is an astonishing thing! You do not know where he comes from, and yet he opened my eyes. We know that God does not listen to sinners, but he does listen to one who worships him and obeys his will. Never since the world began has it been heard that anyone opened the eyes of a person born blind. If this man were not from God, he could do nothing." They answered him, "You were born entirely in sin, and are you trying to teach us?" And they drove him out.

Jesus heard that they had driven him out, and when he found him, he said, "Do you believe in the Son of Man?" He answered, "And who is he, sir? Tell me, so that I may believe in him." Jesus said to him, "You have seen him, and the one speaking with you is he." He said, "Lord, I believe." And he worshiped him. Jesus said, "I came into this world for judgment so that those who do not see may see, and those who do see may become blind." Some of the Pharisees near him heard this and said to him, "Surely we are not blind, are we?" Jesus said to them, "If you were blind, you would not have sin. But now that you say, 'We see,' your sin remains."[1]

The primeval connection between illness and sin resonates so deeply in human experience that even the twenty-first century cannot shake it off. Jesus is asked, "Rabbi, who sinned, this man or his parents, that he was born blind?" And Jesus's reply is startling, "Neither this man nor his parents sinned; he was born blind so that God's work might be revealed in him."

Sin and Illness as Analogous

It is instructive to think about the connection between sin and disease in several ways. One way is by analogy: Just as illness is a disturbance in the physical relationships inside the body (see chapter 3), so sin is a disturbance in spiritual and interpersonal relationships. Illness and sin have at least that much in common. It is also apparent to many clinicians that the brokenness in their patients' bodies often leads them to contemplate the brokenness of their interpersonal relationships. When clinicians say that families can be healed, I think they really mean it. There is a deep sense in which physical restoration and reconciliation are both acts of healing.

Sin as a Causal Factor in Physical Illness

Analogy is not explanation, however. The question I want to explore is not merely whether sin and illness are in any way related, but

whether sin *causes* illness. And in this regard, in some ways this is undeniably true. Medical science does recognize that disturbed interpersonal
relationships can sometimes lead to disturbed psychological states and
that disturbed psychological states may in turn lead to physical illness.
Still, this sort of chain of events is rare and accounts only for a small
proportion of disease and injury. Medical science also is aware that
certain behaviors that religious persons would deem sinful can predispose people to illness. Sexually transmitted disease, for example, would
cease to exist if sexual intercourse were only to occur between mutually
faithful husbands and wives. Yet, although this is true, it is also quite
obvious that much illness and injury occur in the absence of such pre-
disposing sinful behavior. One need not be sinful to be struck by lightning. The perennial question of why bad things happen to good people
reflects the well-known fact that even those who are apparently not
sinners get sick. It is not uncommon to hear a morose intern quip, "He
seems so nice. It must be cancer."

It is difficult to shake the notion that it must be sin that causes
illness—if not the sin of the patient, then that of his parents. Although
later Jewish sources modified the view, the Old Testament supplies
ample scriptural support for such beliefs. God punishes Sodom and Go-
morrah (Gn 19), and even Lot's wife is turned into salt for looking
back (Gn 19:26). The Israelites are promised illness as punishment for
their iniquity. Moses tells them, "The Lord will afflict you with con-
sumption, fever, inflammation" (Dt 28:22). The psalmist prays to God,
like many a patient before and after, saying, "There is no soundness in
my flesh because of your indignation; there is no health in my bones
because of my sin" (Ps 38:3). And Yahweh does tell Moses that punishment does not end with the individual: "For I, the Lord your God, am
a jealous God, punishing children for the iniquity of their parents, to
the third and fourth generation of those who reject me" (Ex 20:5).

It is not uncommon today to hear televangelists declare that certain
illnesses are punishments for certain sins. Yet it is unclear how medically or socially useful it ever is to search for some one-to-one corre-
spondence between a person's illness and some particular sin of that
person or his ancestors. In fact, there is one quick way to refute the
whole notion that illness is divine retribution for particular sins: if sin
causes illness, and everyone sins, then no one should ever be healthy.
Because there are healthy people, however, there must be something
wrong with the premise that all illness is caused by sin.

So the connection between illness and sin must be far more than a mathematical formula. Patients often invoke this erroneous view of the "divine economy," however, thinking that their illnesses are punishments from God. They feel guilty, and clinicians rarely notice or acknowledge their patients' feelings about this. For example, a man may believe that God has punished him with cancer because he put his mother in a nursing home or because he had an affair years ago. Or consider the woman who gives birth to a stillborn child and is sure she did something wrong to cause this. These patients suffer doubly from the anguished belief that the physical illnesses from which they suffer have come about as a punishment for sin.

The idea that there is a causal connection between sin and illness has taken an unprecedented twist in the present era. While the suffering of countless persons continues to be amplified by the view that their illnesses are punishments from God for their personal sins, our narcissistic and litigious society has a new variation on this theme. Many people now seem to think that if they become sick it must be because of someone else's sin—that of McDonald's, or a tobacco company, or their physician. And so they sue. The connection between illness and sin is not just an ancient superstition. It is very much with us today.

The Problem of Finitude

This issue of the relationship between illness and sin must be placed within the larger context of the problem of human suffering. Everyone wants to know why he or she suffers. Yet everyone knows that *everyone* suffers, even if some appear to suffer more than others. Suffering is intrinsic to the human condition. The cup did not pass away from Jesus, and it will not pass away from any of us.

But it pays to look more closely at what we mean by suffering—to think more carefully. Returning to a theme I introduced in the last chapter, I have argued that suffering is always occasioned by human finitude.[2] Suffering is an experience that makes explicit the inherent tension between the intrinsic dignity and the finitude of a person. Pain hurts, but pain becomes suffering only in the moment when one understands how one is limited by it or when it reminds one of one's own ultimate finitude in death.

As creatures, all people are finite—morally, intellectually, and phys-ically. That is to say, people sin, make mistakes, become sick, and die. This is undeniably true. And it cannot be otherwise, for if human be-ings were perfect, they would be gods, not creatures.

Still, although they are finite creatures, human beings have also been endowed by their Creator with the enormous gift of freedom. And if human freedom is to be real, it requires two real possibilities: first, that moral finitude (which is sin) should be a real possibility, and sec-ond, that human beings be capable of choosing not to sin. That is to say, if there is such a thing as freedom, sin and love must both be real possibilities. God has dared to give human beings this freedom. Human beings are *really* free: free to sin and free to love. Thus, if sin were not real, all love would be false.

Paradoxically, however, love can only be concrete if there is real need in the world.[3] If we did not need food, we would never be able to show our love for each other by cooking or eating together. Without the untouchables on the streets of Calcutta, there would be no Mother Teresa. Without sadness, we could not bring joy. Without real human need, there could be no heroes, no saints, no love. The human need that makes the deeds of love possible arises out of our human finitude.

Medicine is one form of real love. Health care professionals can freely minister to the concrete human needs of the finite, embodied persons who present themselves asking for help. Human finitude, in all its forms, occasions medical need. Health care professionals dispose of their freedom in response to this need, and they are free either to sin or to love.

Human intellectual finitude gives rise to medical suffering and need whenever error causes tragedy. For example, a few years ago a piece of metal broke off a poorly designed truck and struck the unsuspecting driver of a car in the opposite lane of a highway. The driver of that car was our hospital's best cardiac surgeon. In a flash, a human error made him a patient and eventually killed him. Patients just like this can show up in any emergency room. Their deepest need is not for someone to blame. They bring their finitude and their need, and they ask their physicians and nurses for love.

Human moral finitude also gives rise to medical suffering and need. Sinful acts do cause illness and injury. Take rape as one horrific exam-ple. A woman who has suffered rape may show up in any gynecology office, bringing her finitude and her need. Certainly there is someone to blame. But such a woman's deepest need is not that her assailant should be convicted and punished by law. In her hour of need she will be asking her physicians and nurses for love.

And finally, human physical finitude also gives rise to that myriad list of human needs that fills the indices of medical textbooks. In the end, no matter how many "causes" are noted for the disease, one will still be left with the question, "And why should that risk factor cause this form of anatomical or physiological malfunction?" The only answer will be the finitude of the human body. The patients who suffer from all these diseases come to health care professionals every day, bringing their finitude and their need. They could, I suppose, mistakenly blame God. But what they are really looking for is love.

So, there is a sense in which St. Paul is right that "the wages of sin is death" (Rom 6:23). But this is not so because of any individual punishment for any individual's sin, but because human sin is *original* in this metaphysical sense—that for there to be real love and real freedom in the world of human beings, sin and death must always have been necessarily real possibilities for human beings. And in the first instance of the human (Adam), the very real possibility of sin became actual. Our history is conditioned by it. We bear it congenitally. We are created with an orientation toward the infinite and an ability to know it (Eden), but the actual world we enter is marked by sin, illness, and death.

This in no way implies that God punishes any individual for his or her sins by making anyone sick. We are created for the infinite, but we are finite as well as free creatures. Our finitude and our freedom entail that both sin and death should be possible. And because we are actual, the possibilities of sin and death are actualized in our concrete lives.

In fact, one might even go so far as to say that for love to become incarnate, death was necessary. For God to show this love for human beings, God had to become human and share in human finitude, embracing even death, death on a cross, conquering both sin and death with his infinite mercy and love (Phil 2:8). In other words, for God's free love to become actual in the finite world of human beings, God's death as a human being was metaphysically necessary. There simply is no real human love without death. Without finitude, the freedom to love cannot be actual. This is the plot of the New Testament, as profound as it is simple: The road to Bethlehem leads inexorably to Calvary. If God really became fully human in the person of Jesus, then

Jesus, as fully human, had to die. There was no other way to show us his love. And so, although "the wages of sin is death," St. Paul finishes his sentence by proclaiming, "But the free Gift of God is eternal life in Christ Jesus our Lord" (Rom 6:23).

Sin, Illness, and the Care of the Patient

As fantastic as it might seem, the ideas discussed in the previous few pages are at the core of what is really going on in the Gospel passage about the man born blind. This passage is about the mysteries of sin and suffering and finitude and freedom and love and incarnation and redemption. This story says simply what is otherwise very complicated to say and very hard to understand. "Go, wash in the Pool of Siloam."

What is perhaps most remarkable, however, is that these exact same mysteries happen every day all over the world in physicians' offices, in clinics, and in hospitals. Each time a sick person comes to a health care professional in finitude and need, the story of the man born blind recurs. Physicians, nurses, and other health care professionals place their hands into the middle of these awesome mysteries every day.

In the story, Jesus does not deny the mystical, metaphysical connection between sin and illness, but he *does* deny that the sin of any individual, family, tribe, or nation has brought illness on anyone as a punishment from God. It is not because of your sin or anyone else's that you are sick, he says, but "that God's works might be revealed in [you]." God's work is love. Healing reveals God's love, and physicians and nurses share in that work of love. Like Jesus, they take up the elements of the earth, the organic and the inorganic, spittle and clay, and they heal. God's works of love are revealed in the midst of the healing professions—in and through the gifts God has given human beings. These gifts include both the elements of the earth and the minds that God has given to those who practice the healing arts. God's healing power comes alive in the world countless times each day in the work of physicians, nurses, and their colleagues—whether through psychoanalysis or hemodialysis; antibiotics or antimitotics; in each EKG and in each PPD.

This is how the wisdom of Ben Sira can come alive again today and nourish those of us who practice the healing arts. As Ben Sira wrote,

"The Lord created medicines out of the earth, and the sensible will not despise them. . . . And he gave skill to human beings, that he might be glorified in his marvelous works. By them, the physician heals and takes away pain; the pharmacist makes a mixture from them. God's works will never be finished; and from him health spreads over all the earth" (Sir 38:4, 6–8).

Physicians, nurses, and other health care professionals desperately need to hear this message today. They need to understand that the suffering of patients is not a punishment for sin, but an opportunity, given to them as health care professionals, for God's glory to be made manifest in their midst. It is tempting (both for politicians looking to lower health care costs and for clinicians) to blame patients, to speak dismissively of them because of the sin they committed that caused them to be ill—cigarette smoking, sexual promiscuity, or, worse, non-compliance with the doctor's orders. It is all too easy to declare certain patients unworthy of time and attention because of the triviality of their complaints. Clinicians sometimes even deem the quality of some of their patients' lives to be so low that in their judgment the "sin" is that these patients are needlessly consuming scarce health resources and time, and so they sometimes dismissively declare them unworthy of both. Judging by what one sometimes hears, one might think that an old adage had been perversely reinvented by health care professionals today: "There but for my own excellent health habits go I."

The hypocrisy of this view should be obvious. Yet, like most self-righteousness, what is obvious is often not apparent to the perpetrators. For instance, I frequently give ethics lectures to house officers who indignantly argue that people who "abuse themselves" by smoking should be refused cardiac bypass surgery. At these noontime lectures, the house officers of whom I speak often have trouble articulating this position because they are actively wolfing down double-cheese pizzas loaded with pepperoni and purchased by pharmaceutical companies that manufacture cholesterol-lowering agents. I ensure that this meal causes them considerable indigestion when I respond that, by their own moral logic, I should refuse *them* cardiac bypass should they need it later in life, given the self-abusive, high-cholesterol eating habits of their youth. Jesus calls us to avoid the trap of blaming the patient and to get on with his work of healing.

Finitude, Illness, and the Community

The foregoing discussion does not imply that health care professionals should not search out the causes of disease and try to change the unhealthy habits of patients. As I will discuss in chapter 10, prevention is good. Human beings ought to be good stewards of their bodies. Nor ought the foregoing discussion be interpreted to mean that health care professionals should not attempt to reduce medical errors. On the contrary, given the certainty of human intellectual finitude, this is a moral imperative. One does need to understand, however, that prevention and quality improvement are different from blaming the patient. In fact, blaming the patient and blaming other health care professionals can be significant barriers to prevention and quality improvement. As a practical matter, patients who are made to feel guilty are less likely to change.

Christians do not deny the reality of sin in the world. The theologian Reinhold Niebuhr once stated that sin is the only theological concept for which there is empirical proof.[4] Nor do Christians deny the reality of intellectual and physical finitude. Christians make mistakes. Christians become sick and die. But if this is the reality that all human beings encounter, however one may choose to try to explain it, these occasions of suffering can be transformed into opportunities for loving action so "that [God] might be glorified in his marvelous works" (Sir 38:6). Illness presents itself as an opportunity for health care professionals to show their love for their brothers and sisters and to learn from those who are ill the valuable lessons they can teach them about faith, hope, and love. Instead, far too often, clinicians communicate, in sometimes subtle ways, that their real attitude toward their patients is that of the Pharisees, who said, "You were born entirely in sin, and are you trying to teach us?" (Jn 9:34).

Patients, through the experience of illness, come to learn the humble truth about their finitude and their radical dependence on God. Such lessons are often hard won and ought *never* to be trivialized. But patients can also be reminded of the service they can provide by teaching the rest of us the invaluable lessons they have learned at the cost of pain. One reason that visiting the sick has always been one of the traditional corporal works of mercy is that it fosters opportunities for the visitors to learn these truths. This is one of the reasons why Catholic Christians bring viaticum from the table of the Lord to the bedsides of patients and celebrate with them the sacrament of the sick. It is not just for the spiritual benefit of the sick, important as this may be. Those who visit the sick should do so as eager students. "Doctor" means "teacher," but the physician is often the patient's pupil.

An Alternate Lesson from the Man Born Blind

Perhaps the greatest lesson health care professionals can take from the Gospel of the man born blind, however, is that they ought not be so quick to identify with Jesus the healer. Physicians and nurses could, easily enough, draw valuable lessons from the story of the man born blind by identifying with Jesus as the healer in the story. But clinicians might learn deeper truths about themselves and about their work if they were to realize that even in their work as physicians, nurses, and other health care professionals, they themselves are men and women born blind. They need to ask Jesus to heal *them*. Physicians and nurses tend to resist this almost instinctually, clinging to their self-conceptions of omniscience and invincibility. Perhaps they say, somewhat pharisaically, "Surely we are not blind, are we?"

But how often have we, as physicians, nurses, and other health care professionals, been blind to the needs of the poor? How often has the crust of greed clouded over our eyes as we pursue privileged lifestyles, indifferent to the needs of the more than forty million U.S. citizens who go without health insurance?

Or how often have we, as physicians, nurses, and other health care professionals, been deaf to the cries of our patients in pain? Have we taken the time to listen to our patients' concerns? Have we dismissed their symptoms? Have we interrupted them with our agendas? Have we cut them off before they have even said what really bothers them?

Or how often have we, as physicians, nurses, and other health care professionals, been mute in the face of the growing immorality of our professions? Officially, our professional societies all promote abortion and increasingly seem to support euthanasia and assisted suicide, the selling of organs, and the commodification of health care. The official voices of our once noble professions seem unable to articulate moral truth.

The process of being healed of one's own professional afflictions will never be easy. But if health care professionals can begin to see themselves as men and women born blind, and if they can bring themselves to ask Jesus to heal them, they might become transformed into the nucleus of a new ministry of healing. Such health care professionals, energized by the Gospel, will doubtless face the wrath of pharisees just as the man born blind did. But if one really has come to understand oneself as someone born blind and now healed, what recourse would one have?

Concluding Prayer

Thus my prayer for my brother and sister physicians is that, like the man born blind,

> You would announce to everyone you see that you have been transformed by his power, even if you do not understand how;
> That you would name him as the one who has healed you;
> That you would go to him.
> And when he asks you, "Do you believe in the Son of Man?" and you find yourself asking, "Who is he, that I may believe in him?"
> That you might recognize the truth of his words when he says, "You have seen him."
> For you have seen him—in eyes yellowed with jaundice and wide as saucers.
> You have heard him—in the cries of the crippled, wondering aloud how God ever allowed this to happen.
> You have touched him—in the bloody wounds of the traumatized.
> (You could have felt the nails if only your own fingers had been healed.)
> You have known the wonder of his presence in the moments of healing that occur over and over again each day, moments in which you have been privileged to share in his healing works.

So when he asks you, say, "Lord, I believe." And worship him. For he *is* what healing means.

CHAPTER 8

Beatitudes

THE Hippocratic-professional synthesis that had been keeping medicine intact as a philosophically coherent enterprise until the end of the twentieth century has now effectively unraveled.[1] In the face of this breakdown, amid the turmoil and the tribulations health care professionals now face, it is only fair to ask what to make of this situation from a spiritual point of view. If one is dispirited, alienated from the task of caring for the sick, longing to see one's work more as a vocation than a job, but frustrated by the various social forces that see it exactly the opposite way, where can one turn?

Although some might think otherwise, academic medicine provides no refuge from this storm. I now dread attending faculty meetings. The only subject we ever discuss is money. We never discuss the quality of patient care, teaching, or research. Most of the physicians who were paid by my hospital to teach have been laid off. The fiscal policy has become, "You eat what you kill: see lots of patients, get big grants, or lose your job. We can no longer afford to subsidize teaching or research at an academic health care center." The tone of conversation is often very bitter. The prevailing attitude among attending physicians at my hospital is disempowerment, bordering on hopelessness.

These attitudes are corroborated by data. Several colleagues and I recently conducted a survey of relatively young physicians who were in practice eight to seventeen years after completing their residency training.[2] Eighty-four percent thought that the traditional ethic of undivided loyalty to patients had diminished in the profession over the last ten years. Fifty-three percent thought their own patients' trust in them had diminished in the last five years. Forty percent were either somewhat dissatisfied or very dissatisfied with their careers.[3]

And now, I fear, my good colleagues in internal medicine are being co-opted. At a faculty practice meeting several years ago, one of my colleagues spoke openly about how she handles telephone calls from patients. She said, "It's very simple. I let the money decide. If they're discounted fee-for-service, I always ask them to make an appointment. If they're capitated, I try very hard to handle everything over the phone." She said this without any apparent trace of shame. What has become of us?

The Beatitudes (Mt 5:1–12) were written for a downtrodden and weary group of Jews who were following a new religious sect that was actively persecuted by the leaders of their traditional religion, in a country occupied by Roman armies that had taxed them into profound poverty. It strikes me that the plight of the audience for the Beatitudes might not be so different from the plight of physicians, nurses, and other health care professionals today. The Beatitudes might have something to say to them.

The First Beatitude

The Beatitudes begin as follows: "Blessed are the poor in spirit, for theirs is the kingdom of heaven" (Mt 5:3). It might not seem that this is an especially resonant note with which to begin. This first beatitude actually seems to distance twenty-first-century health care professionals from the followers of Jesus gathered on that hillside two thousand years ago. Not many physicians are monetarily poor. Some *do* find that their incomes are falling, however, and many are finding that they must see substantially more patients simply to maintain their incomes.[4] A situation of declining income or one in which one is forced to work harder to maintain the same income is never a pleasant situation for any group of laborers. I am sure that it contributes significantly to the presently high levels of physician dissatisfaction. But could this be a blessing? If this beatitude is to be believed, then working harder for the same or fewer real dollars is actually a blessing. That seems like a very strange idea.

How might this downturn in relative income be a blessing to the health professions? One can think of several ways. First, it might chasten the healing professions, forcing them to take a closer, introspective look at what really matters in health care, perhaps even fostering a true

asceticism of practice. Second, the relative downturn in the financial
rewards and lifestyle attractiveness of medicine might draw more people to the profession for the right reasons rather than because an MD
offers more security than an MBA. Third, it might help health professionals to take a wider look around the world, which might make them
more grateful for what they have. With a median net income of
$160,000 per year, even the lowest-paid physicians, those practicing
primary care, are still quite comfortable. If we take the global perspective, it becomes obvious that physician incomes are higher in the
United States than anywhere else in the world, even if they are declining relative to other fields in this country.

But if we put the income question aside, we might find a deeper
spiritual lesson for health care professionals in this beatitude. The
words of St. Francis of Assisi may help to clarify this point: "There are
many who, applying themselves insistently to prayers and good deeds,
engage in much abstinence and mortification of the body, but they are
scandalized and quickly roused to anger by a single word which seems
injurious to their person, or by some other things that might be taken
from them. These persons are not poor in Spirit."[5]

When not just income but also prestige, power, autonomy, and
decision-making authority are taken away, many clinicians have been
scandalized and quickly roused to anger. Physicians do not think of
themselves as blessed these days. That is not what I hear in the doctors'
lounge. I hear anger and indignation. Yet, the spirituality of the Beatitudes says, "Blessed are you."

This does not mean that physicians, nurses, or other health care
professionals should *seek* to be abused and downtrodden. The Beatitudes are not a prescription for masochism. It is a theological mistake
to seek suffering for its own sake. Nor does this beatitude mean that to
live a pious life is to embrace the ultimate form of delayed gratification—suffering now in the hope that God will provide the reward once
one is dead. The words of the Beatitudes are in the present tense:
"Theirs *is* the kingdom of heaven."

What I think this beatitude means for clinicians (and everyone else)
is this: that God is not far from any of us even when we feel impover-
ished, when we lose our money and our power and our prestige, or
when our spirits lag—God is not absent. This is a great and persistent
human temptation—to believe that God is absent when things go

badly and only present when things go well. This belief is understandable, but it is a temptation.

I suspect that many of those working in health care *do* feel powerless
in the face of the changes sweeping their professions. Some of this
change may be good. My own conviction is that much of it is not. But
it may be the case that health care professionals will need to endure a
period of trial and tribulation similar to that of which St. Peter wrote
(1 Pt 1:6–7). This may be so that their faith—in God, in each other,
and in their patients—may be tested like fire-tried gold. All anyone is
ever given is reality—nothing more and nothing less. My brother friar
Richard Rohr, O.F.M., frequently quotes a friend of his as saying, "God
comes to you disguised as your life."6 The Beatitudes say God is there,
in one's life, even when appearances suggest the contrary. One must
engage the surrounding reality as a *spiritual* reality at all times or not at
all. Times of trial and loss are never evidence of the absence of God.
In such poverty of Spirit, letting go of all encumbrances, one finds that
the kingdom is now—even in health care.

The Second Beatitude

The second beatitude states, "Blessed are those who mourn, for they
will be comforted" (Mt 5:4). Scripture scholars suggest that in its original sense this beatitude referred to mourning for the people of Israel—
for the destruction of the Temple that had occurred in the past and for
the destruction that would come soon after the death of Jesus. The
relevance of this reference for medicine became clear to me when I
recalled that I had once participated in a public television documen-
tary titled *The Temple of Science*, which was about the Johns Hopkins
Hospital. The famous dome of the Johns Hopkins Hospital was por-
trayed as that temple. Twentieth-century medicine worshipped at the
temple of science. For many, the dome of the Johns Hopkins Hospital
can still function as a symbol of what they consider to have been the
heyday of medicine—the era of studies in human physiology, of fee-
for-service practice, and of social prestige for physicians. Many physicians have worshipped in that temple, but it is that temple that has
been destroyed. The kingdom of medicine has now been invaded and
occupied by the empire of for-profit biotechnology and the army of the
MBAs. Every pedestal inside the old temple has been knocked down.

Yet, one must remind oneself of the obvious truth that one does not cease to be a physician simply because one's kingdom has been invaded, any more than Jews ceased being Jews when invaded and occupied by Babylonians, Persians, Greeks, or Romans. It is certainly understandable that physicians would mourn the loss of what many consider the golden age of the profession. But this does not mean that the timeless core identity of who and what physicians are has been eradicated. The history of the Hebrew scriptures is one of cycles—destruction, exile, and restoration. Such cycles are also certain for medicine. Golden ages and temples will come and go. There will be a restoration for medicine some day—a new temple in a new form and a new golden era. Some may live to see it; some may not. But if they are to be comforted as the beatitude promises, all those who are in health care because they truly care about patients must remain faithful to their core identity as healing professionals. Moreover, for Christians the real temple and the real golden era belong to the kingdom of God, which although not yet fully instantiated, is already here and now—in the fidelity of God's people and in their proclamation of their own deepest identity.

There will always be patients—sick, vulnerable, frightened—in need of the help that health professionals alone can provide. Physicians, nurses, and other health care professionals can never forget their most fundamental spiritual commitments even as they mourn what has passed. The ultimate hope of the health professions is in the meaning of those commitments.

The Third Beatitude

According to the third beatitude, "Blessed are the meek, for they will inherit the earth" (Mt 5:5). Health care professionals, especially physicians, are not generally thought to be meek. Nevertheless, they have appeared rather powerless to stop what has happened to their professions. Profound changes have occurred in a very short period of time. Physicians especially thought they were very politically powerful, and the public thought so as well. But physicians' own vaunted sense of independence, their confusion about their own identity, their fractiousness, and their self-assurance actually made them easy targets for the major

industrial employers and the insurance companies. In the end, the doctors were pushovers. They wound up divided and conquered. And so
they find themselves knocked back on their heels, reeling, mouths
agape, questioning how so much could have happened so fast with so
little to say on their part. "After all," they ask, "aren't we the experts?"

Again one confronts the ever-paradoxical spirituality of the Beatitudes. Those who are pushed around are called blessed. To apprehend
the meaning of this beatitude requires some reflection. It does not mean
that one should roll over and play dead and simply accept everything
that happens. "Meek" does not mean "naïve" or "weak." It means a way
of relating to other people. It means respectfulness and compassion. It
means that one does not take out one's frustrations on one's patients,
treat utilization reviewers abusively, or storm administrators' offices like
some god out of a Wagnerian opera. Nor does the meekness of the Beatitudes entitle a health care professional to cease being an advocate for
patients. Meekness does not mean moral lassitude.

The Fourth Beatitude

The next beatitude states: "Blessed are those who hunger and thirst
for righteousness, for they will be filled" (Mt 5:6). Most health care
professionals see a great deal of injustice in health care in the United
States today—more than forty million citizens are uninsured, not
counting the undocumented. Those who *are* insured are frequently denied what their physicians think is best for them. And clinicians themselves are also becoming victims of injustice. Some are denied payment
for services they honestly thought were medically justified. Others suffer under the threat of "deselection" by managed care organizations.
The spirituality of the Beatitudes demands that one not turn a blind
eye on such injustice. One must not deny that it exists, attempt to
cover it up, or participate in it.

Wherever health care professionals can do so—humbly, meekly, but
vigorously—they must advocate for justice. They must have a thirst for
justice and seek to quench it. They must recognize that in the current
system patients are frequently treated in the manner described by my
colleague at the faculty practice meeting I discussed earlier in this
chapter. They may be victimized by economic exploitation that will

sometimes cause them to receive more care than is good for them under discounted fee-for-service, and they may be exploited and receive less care than they need when physicians are paid by capitation, bonuses, and withholds. Health care professionals who hunger and thirst for justice will be tireless advocates for justice for their patients, making the extra phone call and enduring the extra paperwork every bit as much as they would endure the inconvenience of answering their pages. Health care professionals who hunger and thirst for justice will also need to become political advocates for patients, doing what they can to make a better system. This is a true asceticism—to endure patiently the hassles and the bureaucratic hardships for the sake of patients. One is not guaranteed the righteousness one seeks. The only righteousness of which one can be sure is one's own capacity to live and to practice justly in the midst of injustice.

God wants mercy, not merely "fasting," from health care professionals today. As Matthew writes, echoing Hosea 6:6, "Go and learn the meaning of the words, 'It is mercy I desire, not sacrifice'" (Mt 9:13). The spirituality of the Beatitudes calls for health care professionals to be merciful and to seek justice for their patients. This is true asceticism. This is the fasting God wants from health professionals.

The Fifth Beatitude

In the fifth beatitude, Jesus says, "Blessed are the merciful, for they will receive mercy" (Mt 5:7). Clinicians have a deep need to forgive themselves, their patients, their government, their nation, and even their insurers. Everyone wants a scapegoat. But it is hard to place blame for the current state of affairs in health care with any precision. Scapegoating is also unnecessary. What the United States needs most is a more merciful health care system.

Mercy is broader than justice. Even while fighting for a more just health care system, physicians and other health care professionals can still learn to be more merciful in their dealings with patients. One way to begin doing so would be to avoid blaming victims. Health care professionals often show little mercy and much hypocrisy when, for instance, they label injection drug users as "self-abusers." (This is a genuinely horrible phrase by which to refer to anyone.) Others would refuse to allow coronary artery bypass grafting in a smoker with progressive angina. Still others expend much energy complaining about the noncompliant patients who (God forgive them!) actually disobey their doctor's instructions.

Mercy is also related to a medical ideal that at first glance might appear to have nothing whatsoever to do with mercy. Since the days of William Osler, the most famous physician of the early twentieth century, clinicians have been urged to cultivate a spirit of *aequanimitas*. This clinical virtue is sometimes misunderstood to mean cold detachment from patients, but as Osler himself actually described it, a clinician's *aequanimitas* springs from the ability to recognize in the patient's foibles at least some foibles not unlike one's own.[7] Thus understood, a*equanimitas* begins to sound a lot like mercy.

In the fullest sense of *aequanimitas*, clinicians also need to be more forgiving of themselves. As the saying goes, "Doctors bury their mistakes." And although this saying is sometimes (unfortunately) literally true, might it also sometimes be figuratively true? Do physicians bury their mistakes deep in their own subconscious minds, finding their humanity and frailty intolerable? What do health care professionals do with the feelings they have when they harm someone seriously through their human negligence and imperfection, especially in a culture that is obsessed with lawsuits? Studies suggest that there is significant psychological stress among clinicians who have made mistakes.[8]

A few years ago, a patient of mine (whom I will call Mr. McCarthy) began to ask me what to do about "floaters."

"Nothing," I replied confidently. "Why do you ask? Are you having floaters?"

"Yes," he said. "A real nuisance."

He was a very nervous sort of patient who, because of his worries about side effects, needed to be coaxed in order to take any medication he needed. I felt good about being able to reassure him. My examination of the inside of his eyes that day was normal.

"Just floaters," I said. "Don't worry."

Two weeks later he called and said: "I'm still worried about these floaters."

"Don't worry," I said. But to reassure him I decided to refer him and said, "Let's have you see the ophthalmologist."

Two months later I found out that his ophthalmology appointment had been set for six weeks after our last conversation. Four weeks before that appointment date, he suffered a retinal detachment.

"New onset dark floaters are harbingers of retinal detachment," the patient told me. "The ophthalmologist told me it was a warning sign that could have saved my vision." He now has 20/200 vision in the affected eye.

This was an awkward moment. I had not known that new onset dark floaters are a vision-threatening sign. As a general internist, this is something I *should* have known. I can assure the reader that I do know it now. It is hardly comforting, however, that the knowledge came at the price of significant visual impairment for one of my patients. Mr. McCarthy specifically expressed his forgiveness toward me. He told me not to worry, that he would not sue me. (I suspect his relatives urged him to sue.) I had not known that there was any kind of floater other than the very common and insignificant type that many patients experience due to opaque spots in the vitreous humor (the clear, gel-like mass between the lens and retina). I had never heard about this more dangerous sign of new onset floaters before anywhere in my education. I now know that they are caused by small bits of blood leaking into the vitreous humor.

I myself needed mercy—from the patient and from God. This was not a "sin" in the sense of a conscious intentional choice to cause harm or some other evil. But it was a manifestation of my own frailty, my humanity, and my weakness. It was just another reminder for me that I am not a god and that I must be careful to forgive my patients for their foibles if I want my own forgiven. This is part of the asceticism of practice—more humbling than a fast. "Blessed are the merciful," says the beatitude. As St. Francis wrote in his own beatitudes, known as the Admonitions, "Where there is mercy and discernment, there is neither excess nor hardness of heart."[9]

The Sixth Beatitude

The sixth beatitude states, "Blessed are the pure in heart, for they will see God" (Mt 5:9). Many kinds of impurity encumber the hearts of people today. Those of us who are physicians, like anyone else, are encumbered by tendencies toward pride, vanity, greed, lust, hurt, fear, cynicism, bitterness, frustration, and guilt.

There is no better way to cleanse the human heart of this sort of accretion than through prayer. I suspect that physicians, nurses, and other health care professionals, who might have an especially great need for prayer, are among the least likely of all professionals to pray on a regular basis. But even in their busyness, they are called to carve out time and space for the silence and the solitude. Only by prayer can one shake off the accretions and recognize the great gap that exists between oneself and the transcendent One who is the source of all healing.

Prayer is a reminder that one is not God, that the healer is also in need of healing and forgiveness. Prayer helps one to focus on what truly matters, helping to cultivate the single-hearted desire to serve one's patients. Prayer helps to strip away the layers of impurity so that God's word can penetrate the heart.

The famous prayer of St. Francis before the crucifix in the ruined church of San Damiano captures this spirit of prayer:

> Most High,
> glorious God,
> enlighten the darkness of my heart
> and give me
> true faith,
> certain hope,
> and perfect charity,
> sense and knowledge,
> Lord,
> that I may carry out
> Your holy and true command.[10]

There are many reasons people practice the healing arts. Some do so for love of science, some for love of money, and some for love of prestige. Some do so because their parents insisted on a medical career. Some do so because after all the years of preparation it would be hard to have done anything else. But only one motive really counts. That motive is the patient.

Almost every human being's motives are mixed, and this is no less true of clinicians' reasons for being in the health care professions. Almost every clinician cares for his or her patients with an imprecise mix of motives—some noble, some not so noble. But in prayer, one's motives can be purified. T. S. Eliot expresses this beautifully in his poem

Four Quartets, in lines that echo the *Showings* of the medieval English mystic Dame Julian of Norwich:

> And all shall be well and
> All manner of thing shall be well
> By the purification of the motive
> In the ground of our beseeching.[11]

With purified motives and chastened hearts, health care professionals will begin to appreciate and give due reverence to the mystery of the patient before them. Prayer helps one to get there—whether meditating, reading scriptures, reciting the rosary, or reflecting while jogging. In prayer, one's otherwise unexamined life undergoes examination—the good parts and the bad parts. Silence exposes the ragged edges of the heart that often only God sees and from which human beings continually attempt to distract themselves. In prayer, the background noise is switched off, so one can finally hear one's most passionate longings echoing deeply, one's most vicious demons snarling angrily, and the voice of God constantly calling one's name.

Health care professionals who learn to hear the leaking valves within their own hearts will learn to hear what is happening inside the chests of their patients in a new way. Such clinicians will learn to practice with a spirit of reverent attention toward their patients. This is the purity of heart to which they are called.

This beatitude promises that if one does all this, one will see God. And this promise is true. One will learn to see God within one's patients. Through prayer and purity of heart one can tear away the veil (cf. 2 Cor 3:12–18) that now separates most clinicians from the innermost meaning of their work. That meaning is the God who dwells inside each patient, for each patient truly is a temple, and each encounter is a pilgrimage to a holy place. Give us clean hearts, O God, that we may see you.

The Seventh Beatitude

According to the seventh beatitude, "Blessed are the peacemakers, for they will be called children of God" (Mt 5:9). My experience is that most health care professionals long to find some semblance of peace in

the frenetic, business-oriented, consumerist, and adversarial atmosphere that dominates contemporary health care. Many sincerely want
to be active agents in bringing peace to their frightened patients and
to their troubled colleagues as well. But most do not know where to
begin. Here is what St. Francis had to say to his own frenetic, business-
oriented, and troubled age: "The servant of God cannot know how
much patience and humility he has within himself as long as everything goes well within him. But when the time comes in which those
who should do him justice do quite the opposite to him, he has only as
much patience and humility as he has on that occasion, and no
more."[12] St. Francis also said, "For the true peacemakers are those who
preserve peace of mind and body for the love of our Lord Jesus Christ,
despite what they suffer in this world."[13]

There is increasing dissension in health care. New payment schemes
now pit generalists against specialists and each against their own.[14]
Under these new financial arrangements, insurance companies contend against hospitals and hospitals against one other. Nurses, nurse
practitioners, and physicians' assistants compete with physicians for
the same limited pool of resources. Far worse, these new financial arrangements pit patients against their physicians and patients against
each other. It is not a kingdom of peace. Everyone feels insecure.
Nurses have long feared (and been victimized by) layoffs. Now physicians share that fear. And patients fear that their genuine needs will
not be met. Everyone is anxious and set on edge. There is a great deal
of rancor in the air. Where can one find peace? How can one make
peace in such a time and place?

Peace can be found, in a situation such as this one, only in fidelity:
fidelity to one's commitments and fidelity to one's patients. Only in
the integrity of doing the right deed for the right reason, and in not
being lured off course by the temptations of greed or cynicism, is peace
possible.

This sort of peace is possible only by way of dispossession. St. Francis
insisted that the early friars would find peace only if they did not have
anything that they could call their own. He said, "If we had possessions
we would need arms for our protection."[15]

No individual health professional owns the medical enterprise. Each
is totally dependent on the work of millions of physicians and nurses
who have gone before and the hundreds of thousands who work together now as a medical community. Today's practitioners were all once

students. When in medical school, or nursing school, or dental school, they did not ask patients for permission to practice on them so that they could then take the knowledge they so gained as their personal, private possession and sell it back to the patients and their children at the highest price the market would bear. No one owns medicine. It is a common heritage. And if one realizes that one does not own it, one will also realize that there is never any reason to resort to force to defend it. Realizing that one does not even own the skills that made it possible to learn the healing arts should make one even more humble. As Ben Sira says (38:1–15), all these gifts ultimately came from God. All any clinician has ever done has been to cooperate with God's healing action. Physicians and nurses would not need to fear that health care would be taken away from them if they were secure in the knowledge that, in the long run, *no one* can ever take possession of health care. It is bigger than every individual practitioner and belongs equally to all practitioners. Any project assuming to the contrary is doomed to fail. The way to peace is a way of dispossession.

The Eighth Beatitude

The final beatitude is perhaps the most relevant for health care today: "Blessed are those who are persecuted for righteousness' sake, for theirs is the kingdom of heaven. Blessed are you when people revile you and persecute you and utter all kinds of evil against you falsely on my account. Rejoice and be glad, for your reward is great in heaven, for in the same way they persecuted the prophets who were before you" (Mt 5:10–12). The average health care professional I know today feels persecuted; these individuals feel hounded by utilization reviewers, strung along by pharmaceutical benefit management companies constantly switching formulary medications, and hounded by patients—especially lawyer-patients—demanding unnecessary care.

But it only takes a moment's reflection to recognize that the profession has weathered worse threats before. After all, doctors and nurses today are only harassed by bureaucrats. Most are not in great danger of contracting tuberculosis or the plague. No one is feeding doctors and nurses to lions.

This may be the spiritual asceticism of practice today—that one must endure the paperwork and the hassles and the constant

CHAPTER 9

The Blood of Christ

*J*UST as there is no single spirituality of marriage, or the priesthood, or work, so there is no single spirituality of health care. Thus far, I have explored various aspects of the spirituality of patients and health care professionals, drawing from scripture, inspirational writings, and my own experience. There is no doubt that this has been a *particular* spirituality—one that has been deeply informed by my own spiritual identity as a Catholic Christian and as a Franciscan. But to some extent I have been holding back. There is no one who has attempted to live the Christian life who inspires me more than St. Francis of Assisi. Although I have quoted St. Francis here and there, I have not tried to articulate anything like a thoroughly Franciscan spirituality of health care. The aim of this chapter is to do just that. These reflections spring explicitly from my own background, experience, reading, prayer, and formation in the Franciscan way of life. Francis is not for everyone. But it is my hope that something from these reflections may be of help even to those readers whose own spiritual journeys will take them in other directions.

Toward a Definition of Franciscan

The first and hardest task in trying to articulate a Franciscan spirituality of health care is to offer a definition of the word "Franciscan." It is not always clear what one means when one describes anything as "Franciscan." One possible (and novel) way to approach a definition of Franciscanism, however, is through the insights of Ludwig Wittgenstein, especially as he is interpreted by Iris Murdoch.[1] Most people recognize that certain things in life really are mysteries, that certain things defy language. According to Wittgenstein, the meaning of these things can only be "shown, not said."[2] The word "Franciscan" seems to point to a reality of just this type. Franciscanism is more easily shown than said. Perhaps Franciscanism belongs to that class of experiences of which T. S. Eliot wrote in the *Four Quartets* when he said, "I can only say, *there* we have been: but I cannot say, where."[3]

The definition of Franciscanism is, in some ways, boundless. Franciscans have a habit of being rather free spirits and extremely inclusive. Yet Franciscanism is not the universe. The boundlessness of Franciscanism is a boundlessness along particular dimensions. One can also err by defining Franciscanism too narrowly—restricting the number of dimensions along which its boundlessness is expressed. This is why a task such as writing a mission statement for a Franciscan health care institution is so hard. I am sure that Francis would laugh and ask, "Mission statement? Don't we have the Gospel?"

Despite all the caveats and risks, however, I would like to propose that there are three specific dimensions of Franciscan compassion that, although not exhaustive of the charism, are at least necessary dimensions of the kind of compassion that would appear to characterize a genuinely Franciscan spirituality in health care. No Christian spirituality of health care will neglect compassion. But Franciscan health care will not be characterized by *generic* compassion. I contend that Franciscan compassion is mediated along at least the following three specific dimensions: Franciscan compassion is personal, incarnational, and imaginative.

By its personal character, I mean that Franciscanism is the most intensely personal of all religious charisms. Francis anthropomorphized the universe. For him, literally everything was personal—he called the sun his brother and the moon his sister. And when Francis described the perfect friar, he listed the names of a dozen friars and their greatest individual virtues—actual persons, not abstract characteristics.[4] For Francis, everything, even death, had the mystery of a person. Like the sun and moon, death was a sibling: Sister Death.

Franciscan spirituality is also incarnational. Francis found God in matter—in the pus of leprous wounds as well as in the word of God as it is proclaimed and preached. As Franciscan theologian St. Bonaventure put it, the light of God is refracted through the matter of the universe, as sunlight pouring through a stained glass window.[5]

According to medieval Franciscan philosopher John Duns Scotus, who developed the principle of individuation known as *haecceitas*, God is found in actual *thisness*.[6]

Franciscan spirituality is also characteristically imaginative. Franciscans insist on the imagination that is necessary for empathy. To understand the suffering of God and the suffering of one's brothers and sisters, as they experience and understand it themselves, requires imagination. One says, in ordinary language, "I can only imagine what you are going through." Compassion requires imagination. The Franciscan charism is highly imaginative—it is dramatic and poetic. Francis dramatically gave his clothes back to his father in front of the bishop of Assisi.[7] Francis also composed the "Canticle of Creatures," the first poem of the emerging Italian idiom.[8] Empathetic, creative, poetic, and dramatic imagination is integral to Franciscan spirituality.

Hagiography and Franciscan Spirituality

As personal, incarnational, and imaginative, Franciscan spirituality, not surprisingly, is inherently hagiographic—the personal stories of real people who live the charism. For Franciscans, spirituality is biography—Francis and Clare, Anthony and Agnes, Bernadine and Margaret: shown, not said.

Consequently, Franciscan spirituality is essentially without method. There is no prescribed pattern. There are no exercises. To be a person is not to follow a method. Persons live concrete historical lives and concrete spiritual lives. There is no essential difference between the two.

And so to explore a spirituality of health care in the Franciscan tradition, one must first turn to the story of this person named Francis. There is no other way. Because the story of Francis is too long to tell in all its rich detail, I will undertake this task by looking at four points in his life in which Francis confronted sickness and death—his own and that of others. These are highly significant points in his biography, suggesting that the encounter with sickness and death is not peripheral to the Franciscan story. These four nodal points are his early illness, his embracing of the leper, his experience on Mount Alvernia, and his own death. I will look to each of these nodal points to establish that the personal, the incarnational, and the imaginative are distinctively

Franciscan elements of the compassion in each of these events. From these stories I will distill lessons for a Franciscan spirituality of health care.

FRANCIS'S EARLY ILLNESSES

As the story is most charitably told, Francis seems to have spent a happy-go-lucky youth. He lived in turbulent times, however. Francis appears to have fought in the bloody 1202 war between the city states of Perugia and Assisi and may even have been taken prisoner.[9] Somewhere around this time, he "was worn down by his long illness," and he began "to mull over within himself things that were not usual for him."[10] As Bonaventure noted in describing this period in Francis's life, "Affliction can enlighten spiritual awareness."[11] Health care professionals perhaps need little reminding of the ways in which serious illness seems to clarify what is important for people, the way it tests, purifies, and teaches. Francis, it seems, learned these lessons at a young age. And a "divine fire on the inside" began to warm his youthful blood.[12]

What exactly happened to him during this illness? The biographies provide no details. But whatever happened, this much is sure: Francis began to change. His youth had been bent by a wintry fever.[13] And his first recorded act after this illness was an act of compassion for a poor knight. The biographies note the very personal character of the compassion of Francis. He apparently felt for the knight because this poorly dressed man was of noble birth but had fallen on hard times. Francis understood instantly and keenly the knight's personal story and his suffering. Only a sensitive person understands the embarrassment of another. The compassion of Francis was immediately concrete. His first response was to take care of the knight's physical needs—to relieve his poverty. With characteristic imagination, he gave the knight his cloak. This was a broad and dramatic gesture—at once an act of compassion and a lesson for all to see.

Shortly thereafter, still uncertain about what was happening to him, Francis had a dream in which he saw shields emblazoned with a red sign of the cross.[14] He did not know it then, but the red cross depicted on those shields would drive his red blood from that moment until the end of his life. Francis's compassion was marked by the sign of the cross before he ever understood it.

Embracing the Leper

As Francis's conversion continued to unfold, the next nodal point along the way was his encounter with a leper. As he himself would later say, "And the Lord led me among [lepers] and I showed mercy to them."[15] He felt compassion for them in the blood and the pus of their wounds. As Bonaventure said of the compassion of Francis, "It was through this virtue that he was attracted to all redeemed in the blood of Christ."[16]

His compassion for the leper was characteristically personal—horror and revulsion gave way to an interpersonal relationship. The object of his fear became the subject of his love. And he showed this compassion in characteristically incarnational ways—he gave the leper an alms, then kissed him on his festering cheek. Readers sometimes miss the fact that Francis cared for the leper's needs before he kissed him. Incarnational Franciscan compassion is preeminently practical.

And Francis's compassion for the leper was also overwhelmingly imaginative. Francis had the imagination to see that the call to "knighthood" about which he had dreamed would be accomplished through the discipline and training that would give him the courage to love. He had the imagination to see in the alienation of the leper his own alienation and the alienation of Christ.

In the leper, Francis saw Christ crucified, and he reached out to him in compassion. Francis embraced the leper "because of Christ crucified, who according to the text of the prophet was despised as a leper."[17] He saw in the alienation of this stranger's dust the strangeness of his own dust and the strangeness of the dust that Christ took on out of love for all humankind.

And shortly thereafter, Francis heard the voice of the Crucified One speak to him in the church of San Damiano. Francis must have spent a long time staring at that crucifix. He must have noticed that the wounds of Christ, as depicted on that crucifix, are represented as fountainheads that are sprinkling blood on the angels and the saints. These were the wounds Francis saw in the wounds of the leper. As his understanding of his vocation grew, he would one day understand that the command he heard from the Christ of San Damiano to "re-build the church" had nothing to do with bricks but "was really about that Church which Christ acquired with his own blood."[18] The cross of Christ is the living sign of love—the open-handed, unclenched love that needs no armaments and the silk and rough love that breaks all rocks, splits boulders in two, and quakes the living earth.[19] Francis felt it in himself and in the leper.

MOUNT ALVERNIA

Many years later, Francis's compassion for the Crucified One would reach a height unparalleled in Christian discipleship. While meditating atop Mount Alvernia, Francis saw a six-winged seraph appear before him, nailed to a cross. "The fact that [the seraph] was fashioned to a cross pierced his soul with a sword of compassionate sorrow."[20]

Francis actually had compassion for Christ. Who else could claim such a personal, intimate relationship with God? Who could actually claim compassion for the living God from whom every human being must so constantly *seek* compassion? "By his sweet compassion he was being transformed into him who chose to be crucified because of the excess of his love."[21]

The compassion of Francis reached out to Christ in the flesh. And Francis felt that compassion so intensely that the compassion of Christ became incarnate in him. The compassion Francis felt for Christ was so real that it burned his flesh. "Sacred" blood began to flow from his wounded side.[22] "It represent[ed] to the eyes of faith that mystery in which the blood of the spotless lamb, flowing abundantly through the five wounds, washed away the sins of the world."[23]

And the compassion of Francis for the crucified Christ was also imaginative. Francis encountered the suffering of Christ in the form of a six-winged seraph. Francis's imagination was sufficiently expansive that he could identify with the suffering of Christ to the point of bearing the brand marks of Christ in his own body.

The compassion Francis showed (and was shown) on Mount Alvernia challenges our imaginations. From the thirteenth to the eighteenth centuries, this mysterious event became, aside from the Crucifixion, the Nativity, and the Madonna and Child, perhaps the most frequently depicted subject in Western art. Giotto, Fra Angelico, Bellini, van Eyck, Caravaggio, El Greco, Rubens, and dozens of other masters all strained their artistic imaginations in trying to capture on canvas St. Francis receiving the stigmata. Perhaps because the event is far more easily shown than said, fewer poets have dared to try to capture in words what Alvernia was like. Even Dante left us only three brief (if beautiful) lines:

> nel crudo sasso intra Tevero e Arno
> da Cristo prese l'ultimo sigillo,
> che le sue membra due anni portarno.
>
> [On that barren rock between the Tiber and the Arno
> Where Christ pressed into his flesh that final and decisive seal
> He would carry in his members for his last two living years.][24]

Franciscan compassion is lived in blood and in the cross. It is not placebo compassion. It is not "feel-good" religion. Yet Franciscan compassion is also never dour. To enter into the pain of another is the path to eternal bliss. Francis Thompson understood this when he called the stigmata of St. Francis "wine-smears on thy hand and foot."[25] The blood of absolute compassion is the wine of perfect joy. Franciscan compassion is unto eternal life, born of the conviction that such a life became real in the person of Jesus.

Sister Death

Having embraced Christ crucified with such love, Francis turned finally to face his own death. The death of St. Francis has been highly romanticized, but it was, in fact, quite gruesome. He vomited blood.[26] The wound on his side bled continuously. It caused the brothers to "remember the One who poured out blood and water from his own side and reconciled the world to the Father."[27]

Francis's relationship with death was so remarkably intimate and personal that he called death his "sister."[28]

> Laudato si, mi signore, per sora nostra
> morte corporale,
> da laquale nullu homo
> vivente po skappare.
> Guai acqueli ke morrano
> ne le peccata mortali!
> Beati quelli ke trovarane
> le tue santissime voluntati,

ka la morte secunda
nol farà male.

[Praise be you, my Lord, through Sister Death,
From whose embrace no mortal can escape.
Woe to those who die in mortal sin.
Happy those She finds doing your will.
The second death will do them no harm.][29]

Francis's death was a highly interpersonal event. He encountered death as a relationship. He died surrounded by persons who loved him—the friars, St. Clare, and his friend and patroness, Lady Jacoba. He embraced life as well as death even as he lay dying.

Francis's death was also profoundly incarnational. He insisted that he be placed naked on the ground. Yet the great ascetic received cookies from Lady Jacoba as he was dying.[30] He had a craving, as the dying often have, like the craving of a pregnant woman. He was about to be born into the next life, naked as he had entered this one.

Finally, the death of Francis was imaginative. Francis staged a paraliturgical feast before he died. He could identify so much with his living Savior that he broke bread with him and his disciples and discoursed at length about his love.

Those who would bear witness to this death and claim to draw inspiration from it would do well to contemplate Francis's attitudes of intimacy and praise. Francis is no longer with us in body, but his death abides with us still in the flesh of this world, for deep with the first dead lies Assisi's son. After the first death, there is no other.[31]

In his dying, Francis showed other Christians how to die and how to care for the dying: "Living, to imitate Christ living, dying, to imitate Christ dying, and after death to imitate Christ after death."[32] "In all things, he wished to be conformed to Christ crucified, who hung upon the cross poor, suffering, and naked."[33] He strove to teach all persons to love God and to love all other persons with this deep sort of compassion—personal, incarnational, and imaginative. Of the friars who saw his sacred stigmata for the first time as he lay dying, Celano wrote, "Whose heart would be so much like stone that it would not break with sorrow, that it would not burn with divine love, or would not be strengthened with good will?"[34]

Franciscan Spirituality and Health Care

What does all of this mean for those who care for the sick? I would argue that Franciscan health care must be informed by this same spirit of compassion: one that is personal, incarnational, and imaginative. This means that a Franciscan spirituality of health care must be sealed in blood, marked by the sign of the cross. For Francis, the logic was simple. God is a person. God's imaginative compassion for his creatures took flesh in the person of Jesus. And in the imaginative spiritual theology of Franciscanism, once one really understands the meaning of the Incarnation—that Jesus was one person, fully human and fully divine—the Paschal Mystery becomes a mere deduction. As human he had to die, and as divine he had to rise. And so the meaning of the personal, the meaning of the incarnational, and the meaning of the imaginative meet at the foot of the cross. In the logic of Franciscan spirituality, it then becomes obvious that following the compassionate way of the cross is the only sure way to salvation. The cross was the one sign that Francis saw throughout his life—marking the shields of his youthful sickbed dreams, marking the illness of the leper, marking his own body on Alvernia, and, finally, marking his death. In Franciscan spirituality, all are redeemed through the cross of Christ, the visible sign of God's love. All are redeemed as persons by a God who is personal, became incarnate for us, and gives us the imagination to hope in the love that heals us.

As the Gospels tell it, the physical suffering of Christ is concentrated into a period of less than twenty-four hours. This is a remarkable point on which Christian health care professionals can meditate fruitfully, believing that everything any patient (or any health care professional) will ever suffer is subsumed in a historical drama that unfolded in less than a day. Francis understood this drama and its power. He saw it in the San Damiano crucifix. He saw it in his dreams. He saw it in the leper. He saw it in his own suffering and in his own death.

And so, a Franciscan spirituality of health care must be marked by a compassion that is as deeply personal as the Passion of Christ. Every patient's ordeal is the story of a person, and this story must be linked with the story of the person of Christ.

Marked by its incarnational emphasis, Franciscan spirituality will always recognize that illness is a spiritual as well as a physical event.

The Word became flesh. Afflictions of the flesh can enlighten spiritual awareness in anyone, just as the early illness of Francis awakened his spiritual life. Human persons are constituted as body and spirit at once, and illness grasps human beings as whole persons.

Marked by its imaginative emphasis, a Franciscan approach to health care can never be mere bioengineering. It must engage patients as persons, endowed not only with the dignity that comes from having been created in the image and the likeness of God but also with the alien dignity that comes from having been redeemed by the cross of Christ.[35] A genuinely Franciscan spirituality of health care does not treat patients as mere isolated organs or as mere consumers of health care resources. Rich or poor, young or old, citizen or alien, able or disabled, the personal in every person is boundless and of inestimable worth. A practitioner imbued with a Franciscan spirituality will even be imaginative enough to be aware of the embarrassment that patients often feel, just as Francis understood the embarrassment of the poor knight. Practitioners imbued with the Franciscan spirit will recognize how the sick are often shunned. They will move past any initial hesitation or revulsion and reach out to touch their patients personally, as Francis embraced the leper. Practitioners imbued with the Franciscan spirit will understand the essential unity of their own suffering and the suffering of Christ. They will be able to feel the suffering Christ in their own persons. They will find unity with his suffering through active engagement with their own suffering and that of their patients, just as Francis did on Alvernia. And they know that they can truly minister to the needs of the dying only if they can learn to call death their sister.

Compassion of this sort can only be shown, not said. It is the compassion of Francis and Clare. It is the compassion spoken of by Mother Alfred Moes, foundress of the Franciscan Sisters of Rochester, Minnesota, who gave the father of the famous Mayo brothers the idea to start a hospital that would be staffed by her sisters. She told Dr. William Worrell Mayo, "The cause of suffering humanity knows no religion or sex; the charity of the Sisters of Saint Francis is as broad as their religion."[36]

A Franciscan spirituality of health care must also demonstrate incarnational compassion, which means compassionate action. The most tender stories of Francis and Clare concern their personal care and solicitude for the sick brothers and sisters of their orders. Austerity was always tempered with concrete compassion. The plight of the sick led Francis and Clare to relax fasts, feed grapes to the sick, and provide feather pillows and wool blankets to their confreres experiencing physical discomfort.[37]

Incarnational compassion means emptying bedpans. It means using morphine amply yet judiciously to relieve the pain of dying patients. It means binding patients' wounds with reverence and love. And it means taking the time to listen, even as time becomes increasingly scarce. Health care professionals who live a Franciscan spirituality will be present to their patients in the flesh.

Incarnational compassion also demands working for justice in health care. Francis gave the leper an alms before he kissed him. Incarnational compassion means going the extra mile to fight for the needs of patients when they are denied essential care by the new merchant class that is now transforming health care the way the thirteenth-century merchant class transformed the Europe of St. Francis. Incarnational compassion means working to change a system that, by denying them health insurance, has exiled more than forty million Americans outside the walls of the medical city-state. Incarnational compassion means preaching the Gospel of Life to a society marked by violence—toward the unborn, toward enemies in foreign lands, toward prisoners on death row.[38]

A Franciscan spirituality of health care will also be imaginative. Practitioners with genuinely Franciscan imagination see in the suffering of patients, and in their own suffering, the suffering of Christ the Lord. Francis believed he had a duty toward the sick and the poor because he always saw in them the image of Christ, poor and suffering.[39]

The world is suffused with suffering. Doctors, nurses, psychologists, and other health care professionals know this better than anyone else. They are capable of learning to identify with that suffering. The world is our wound.[40] Like the friars at the deathbed of Francis, health care professionals put their hands into the bloody wound of human suffering every day. Health care professionals must have the religious imagination to find God there. At the tip of the spleen, at the point of the knife, at the rising mercury's edge—God is in the suffering and in the compassionate hand that reaches out with healing.

A Franciscan spirit of imagination will also encourage and engage in scientific research for the sake of the sick. Franciscan spirituality is not anti-intellectual or anti-scientific. All those who wear glasses or contact lenses can thank Friar Roger Bacon for his pioneering work in optics. Finding cures for diseases through research and imagining new ways to ameliorate the symptoms of those who are suffering are preeminently Franciscan activities. To do so is to work creatively with the gifts God has given humankind through our sister Mother Earth and through the exercise of God's gifts of reason and imagination. Lady Jacoba made cookies. Perhaps a Franciscan of the twenty-first century will discover a new pharmaceutical agent to treat Alzheimer's disease.

Franciscan imagination will also challenge health care professionals to create new health care structures. Perhaps the command of the crucified Christ of San Damiano speaks most loudly to health care professionals today by urging them to rebuild the house of health care, which is surely falling into ruins. Health care today is increasingly impersonal. Health care today increasingly replaces the incarnational aspects of care with machines. Health care today increasingly dulls the imagination, turning patient care into an assembly line. Health care today seems increasingly devoid of compassion, drowning out the desperate cries of the sick and poor with tired old mantras about cost control and the need to avoid the evils of socialized medicine. As Francis said, "Go and repair my house, which, as you can see, is falling completely into ruin."[41]

In the Spirit of the Blood of Christ

Francis saw in the suffering of others the suffering of Christ. He engaged them with a compassion that was personal, incarnational, and imaginative. He saw all around him a people redeemed by the blood of Christ. He saw in the blood that flowed from the five wounds of the Crucified One of San Damiano a fountain that bathes and redeems all people. The blood of Christ made the blood of Francis shake. But one should never forget that the blood of a leper also made the blood of Francis shake—for the sake of the blood of Christ. Just so, the blood of our wounded brothers and sisters—the ones we see in our hospitals and offices every day—ought now to make our own blood shake for the sake of the blood of Christ.

In the care of our patients, we stand daily at the foot of the cross. "God's Mary in her grief."[42] The blood of Christ, the blood of Francis, the blood of the leper, the blood of our patients, and our own blood are all one. For "the cup of blessing that we bless, is it not a sharing in the blood of Christ?" (1 Cor 10:16).

It is worth noting that Francis almost never said "communion" when he referred to the Eucharist. Consistently personal, incarnational, and imaginative, Francis always said we receive "the Body and Blood of Christ."[43] These days, when it has almost become a cliché to say that one's spirituality is "incarnational," Franciscan spirituality must recognize that this means real blood.

Thomas of Celano said that the followers of Francis—the Poverello—the glorious poor one of Christ— would remain vital and strong "as long as the blood of the poor Crucified was warm in their memory and the wonderful cup of his suffering inebriated their hearts."[44] This is our challenge in health care today: to follow the course of the blood that ran through the veins of Francis; to practice our healing professions in a way that is shown, not said, and lived, not recited; to practice in a way that is personal, incarnational, and imaginative; to render compassionate care in the blood of Christ. This is the Gospel way Francis showed us. May God show each of us which way is our own.

chapter 10

The Temple of the Holy Spirit

*I*N this chapter I will turn from considering the spirituality of caring for the sick human body to considering the spirituality of caring for the healthy human body. I will begin my explorations with a simple question. What if people were to take seriously the notion of St. Paul (1 Cor 6:19) that the human body is the temple of the Holy Spirit? Too often, this phrase is recited glibly and its meaning easily missed. If one considers St. Paul's words seriously, however, the meaning may be surprising.

A temple is a sacred space. The idea of a sacred space may be novel for those who dwell in the cities and suburbs of the twenty-first-century Western world, even for those who call themselves Christian. Accordingly, some explanation is in order. Although God is truly present everywhere, anthropologists and historians of religion point out that for the religious person, God is present in certain spaces in a qualitatively different way.[1] Whenever God's presence becomes manifest to human beings in some important, startling, or new way, *homo religiosus* (Mircea Eliade's technical term for human beings as intrinsically religious creatures) calls the place where this has occurred "sacred." These sacred spaces may be almost anywhere, but often they are places of natural beauty—along a shore, at a waterfall deep in the woods, or on a mountaintop. They may be places that have profound historico-spiritual significance, such as Ground Zero after September 11, 2001. They may be places that hold a special significance in one's religious heritage, such as Bethlehem or Gethsemane for Christians and Mecca for Muslims. They may be places where miracles have happened, such as Lourdes. They may simply be places designated for worship, places that house the faithful who have gathered to give thanks and praise to God, places that safeguard sacred words and rituals. From time immemorial, human beings have erected altars in the locations they consider sacred—where God has been experienced in a profound way.

So what St. Paul seems to be saying is that all of this is also true of the human body. After all, it is in human bodies that worship happens. It is in human bodies that the words and rituals of our religion are safeguarded. It is in human bodies that all the historico-spiritual events of Christianity have taken place. Most important, Christians believe that God's self-revelation took place succinctly and completely in the human body of the Incarnate Word, Jesus Christ. The human body is a sacred space.

The human body is the place where human life and human love happen. The crafts of medicine, nursing, dentistry, and all the other healing arts require at least two human bodies—that of the healer and that of the one who is healed. It is in human bodies that the spirit of God transforms the air we merely breathe into the grace of God that touches every cell in our mortal bodies, forms any words of Good News we will ever proclaim, and moves us to works of charity and worship.

Sometimes, however, St. Paul is taken to have a different view of the body. St. Paul is frequently misinterpreted as advocating that we should hate our bodies. Admittedly, a few passages in the Pauline epistles might suggest such an interpretation. He writes, for instance, "We know that our old self was crucified with him so that the body of sin might be destroyed, and we might no longer be enslaved to sin" (Rom 6:6). He also makes such comments as, "For this reason the mind that is set on the flesh is hostile to God; it does not submit to God's law—indeed it cannot, and those who are in the flesh cannot please God" (Rom 8:7–8). But St. Paul never says that one should hate one's body. In fact, in Ephesians 5:29, in discussing the relationship between husbands and wives, noting that the two are one flesh, he declares, "For no one ever hates his own body, but he nourishes and tenderly cares for it, just as Christ does for the church."

Although there are undeniable elements of Greek dualism in his writings, St. Paul's use of the term "flesh" can generally be read as shorthand for excessive attention to bodily pleasure. St. Augustine, after citing this passage from St. Paul's Letter to the Ephesians, notes:

> Man, therefore, ought to be taught the due measure of loving, that is, in what measure he may love himself so as to be of service to himself. For

that he does love himself, and does desire to do good to himself, nobody but a fool would doubt. He is to be taught, too, in what measure to love his body, so as to care for it wisely and within due limits. For it is equally manifest that he loves his body also, and desires to keep it safe and sound. And yet a man may have something that he loves better than the safety and soundness of his body.[2]

Augustine is saying that it is natural, normal, and healthy to love one's body. But when one loves one's body in a proper way it is because one first loves one's whole self in a proper way, and one's self is not reducible to one's body. What can one love better than the safety and soundness of one's body? First and foremost, Augustine suggests, one must love one's whole self. As an embodied person, one's personhood is not reducible to the body. One's body deserves love in "due measure." More love of the body itself than this threatens to become the love of the flesh that is hostile to God and God's plan for each human being.

St. Paul emphatically dismisses the view that the body is an evil prison in which the true human being is trapped. The body is a temple, and a temple is not evil. To caution, as Paul does, against the wanton use of one's body is not to say that the body is evil. Understanding one's body to be a temple means that it is good. After calling the body the temple of the Holy Spirit, St. Paul goes on to urge that one "glorify God in [one's] body" (1 Cor 6:20). Yet this same understanding carries with it certain undeniable responsibilities.

The first of these responsibilities is gratitude. God has given each human being a body. We are embodied creatures. This is the kind of thing we are. The gift God has given us in our bodies is thoroughly amazing. Far too often we take it for granted and forget to give thanks for this gift. Each body, as the scriptures say, is "fearfully and wonderfully made" (Ps 139:14). No matter how much one might think one's body less "perfect" than that of the idealized Greek god or goddess, each human body *is* fearfully and wonderfully made. Health care professionals know this from the inside out.

Human bodies are good. God has said so. In the Book of Genesis (1:31), God pronounces all that he has made to be "very good." The truly reflective person is compelled to stand in awe at the marvel and the mystery of who she or he really is as a fully embodied person. Health care professionals can count the ability to arrive at this perspective as one of the great privileges of their work. Having studied the inner workings of the human body in great detail, they are poised to stand in awe at the marvel and the mystery of the embodied human person.

Sometimes, it is true, physicians and other health care professionals can almost delude themselves into thinking that *they* are the creators, not God. But "M.D." does not stand for "medical deity" no matter what any physician may actually think or say to the contrary. Sometimes health care professionals can deny or suppress the incredible mystery that presents itself in the glimpses they have of the complex workings of the human body. That human beings exist at all, that human beings were created by God in such an intricate and wonderful way, that the human body grows, and that it heals itself all ought to be occasions for praise.

No matter what medical scientists ever do in the laboratory—after they have sequenced every last strand of DNA—they will not be able to tell any human being what it really means to be human. We are *not* our genes. The mystery of the human mode of being is the unseen axis about which the double-helix of human DNA is coiled. The human mode of being cannot be seen under a microscope or displayed as a pattern of DNA fragments arrayed on a gel. Human beings are made in God's own image and likeness (Gn 1:26). God calls human beings his children, a title of affection that God does not even bestow on the angels.

Human beings are subject to the laws of genetics, it is true. But to say this is to say very little about the *meaning* of human genetics. Through our genes, we carry the lives of our great-grandparents and their great-grandparents—right in the cells of our marrow, livers, and brains. Our forbearers are still with us—a bit of Abraham in every Jew and a bit of Adam in all of us. Through the families that raised us, we were also given nurturance and the space to grow. And it is God who has given us both—the wonders of nature and the wonders of nurture—here and now.

In fact, Christians believe God actually loves each member of the human race so much that he became human—taking on flesh and taking on a body like that of any other human being. Jesus was not a ghost temporarily renting a human body. Jesus ate, drank, sweated, breathed, and felt pain and pleasure just like any other human being who has ever lived.

The goodness of the human body is so profound that the human body of Jesus still nourishes his children down to this very day—every day—in the Eucharist. Jesus gives his followers the goodness of his body.

Our own bodies are good. They are great gifts. Sometimes one only needs to pause to reflect on the obvious. Breathing is amazing. Seeing is amazing. Hearing is amazing. Healing is amazing. Each human being should be grateful to God for the gift of his or her body and ought to be careful to dispose of such a great gift in a manner befitting its beauty, its dignity, and its value.

Stewardship of the Body

Each human being, then, can legitimately be considered the rector of a cathedral—the person in charge of a sacred space. That sacred space is his or her body. Each must also be reminded that being in charge of a temple requires certain virtues. One must maintain a spirit of reverence and awe. One must be sure that the space is not used for illegitimate purposes that might profane its sacred character. And one must treat it with care and respect and be sure to attend to its upkeep.

This means that believing Christians should take good care of their bodies. This is not just a polite suggestion echoing the advice mothers have given their children throughout the centuries. All believers have a very significant Christian duty to be good stewards of their bodies.

Stewardship is a word often associated with parish finances. The Stewardship Committee is the congregation's finance committee. But the basic concept of stewardship is broader. The theme of stewardship in the Gospel parables is that just as those who are good stewards of property and finances will be rewarded by their masters, so will God reward those who are good stewards of the religious bequest they have been given. The central thesis of this chapter is that the Lord God asks all people to be good stewards of the bodily bequest they have been given as well.

A good steward does not squander what has been put in his or her charge. A good steward does what is required for the upkeep of the estate and does not begin "to eat and get drunk" (Lk 12:45) instead. A good steward makes sure that the master's investment does not remain static but grows and develops in a healthy way (Mt 25:14–30). The same is true of the human body. Given such a great gift, human beings are duty bound to be sure that it is nurtured and that it develops in a healthy way.

Taking proper care of one's body is not selfish or vain. Healthy and proper attention to one's body is a discipline of gratitude and charity. There are many pure and holy motives for caring for one's body. One can care for one's body out of gratitude to God. One can care for one's body so that one may remain healthy enough to offer praise to God. And one can care for one's body so as to remain fit enough to attend to the material needs of one's brothers and sisters.

So, the proper Christian motive for preventive medicine is steward-ship of the body, that is, the upkeep of a sacred space. This is why one should be screened for cancers with tests that have been shown effec-tive in preventing premature death due to cancer, why one should be vaccinated against pneumococcal pneumonia when one reaches sixty-five years of age, and why one should have regular blood pressure checks and be screened for high cholesterol. The body is a temple of the Holy Spirit. With such a tenant, deferred maintenance is not an option.

Responsible stewardship is balanced, however. One ought not to go overboard. Having a body is like having a cathedral under one's charge. One should not let the cathedral decay with neglect. But neither should one spend enormous time and effort polishing every square cen-timeter of brass and marble in the place and then refuse to let anyone enter to make use of it. Good stewardship means responsible care for one's body—not being wanton and reckless, not being neglectful, and not being miserly or afraid to share it.

Prodigality

The very same scripture story that I used in chapter 5 to discuss the state of the medical profession today—the story of the prodigal son—can also help to illuminate a common problem in contemporary West-ern society's relationship with the human body. First, however, one needs to be clear about what this strange word, "prodigal," actually means. I would be willing to wager that less than 5 percent of high school students taking the Scholastic Assessment Test could define it. Perhaps it merely sounds familiar because of its attachment to this Gos-pel story.

The dictionary defines "prodigal" as meaning reckless and wasteful. Someone who is prodigal is someone who does not take care of the good things he or she has been given, but wantonly abuses and squanders them all. This is what the prodigal son did with his father's fortune. He wantonly abused his patrimony and squandered it all on dissolute living. The opposite of being prodigal is being a faithful steward of one's fortune—taking care of and nurturing the goods one has been given.

Human beings can be prodigal about their bodies in two ways. First, one can become wanton and reckless and lead a life dominated by the pursuit of bodily pleasure. Everyone probably knows at least some of these people. All of us have had our own "prodigal moments." But those who suffer from the vice of prodigality are habitually predisposed to such prodigal moments. They reel about between the cocktail hour and the coffee bar. For some, taking marriage vows is seen as an unnecessary restriction on their freedom to pursue sexual pleasure. For others, the vows are taken but trivialized. Witness the recent marriage of a pop-music star, lasting all of fifty hours, undertaken as a lark, a joke, a dare. Prodigal persons are overfed, oversexed, or both. The old-fashioned names for these sins are gluttony and lust. Today, even the idea that it is possible to be gluttonous or lustful is derided sarcastically, dismissed by our society as anachronistic. But these sins are old-fashioned only in name. In fact, they are with us just as deeply as ever. Sometimes, sadly, they are put on display in a very public fashion. More often, they are indulged in much more subtle ways. The pursuit of the perfect bottle of wine and the search for even more haute cuisine are common forms. Perhaps even more common today is the person who professes that curious form of fidelity that takes shape as serial monogamy—never more than one sexual partner at a time, but no partner for more than one year. Each "relationship" is driven only by sex, until the thrill is gone, and each passes on to the next, short-lived "relationship."

The advice given in the Book of Sirach (37:27–31) is still a wise corrective for the excesses of our own age:

> My child, test yourself while you live; see what is bad and do not give in to it.
> For not everything is good for everyone, and no one enjoys everything.

Do not be greedy for delicacy, and do not eat without restraint;
For overeating brings sickness, and gluttony leads to nausea.
Many have died of gluttony, but the one who guards against it
prolongs his life.

It is not hard to imagine how these forms of prodigality can ruin the temple, destroying its structure along with the spirit within. Perhaps the most important public health epidemic in the United States today is obesity.[3] Rather than restraining behavior, patients prefer pills so they can continue to pursue unlimited gastronomic pleasure without ill effects on their health. Some seem to think this is a birthright. Astonishingly, the success of certain drugs in the treatment of HIV infection has led some, whose lust was only temporarily mitigated by fear, to revert to hyperpromiscuous behavior. Concomitantly, public health officials have noted rises in new cases of syphilis, gonorrhea, and, most horrifying of all, HIV.[4] The purpose of medicine is viewed by some almost as an instrument for enabling morally, spiritually, and physically unhealthy living rather than a craft for coaxing imbalanced and disordered bodies back into equilibrium.

The second way human beings can be prodigal about their bodies is to pay excessive attention to their health. For some people, the golden calf they worship is their own health. This is a very subtle but increasingly common problem. It is not exactly vanity but a variation on prodigality. It passes for discipline or even asceticism. But it is a trap in which many people seem to have become ensnared.

Everyone also knows this sort of person. The language people sometimes use betrays the frequently twisted priorities of the twenty-first century. These days, the only thing anyone is willing to call decadent is chocolate cake. "No, I couldn't. That would just be decadent."

It does not seem to matter with whom one has had sex, or how many lies one has told, or whose life one has ruined in the pursuit of a successful career. For these people, it is cholesterol-laden bacon and eggs that are obscene, and it is the failure to get to the health club that represents moral laxity. Such persons eat all the right organic foods, jog, lift weights, floss their teeth twice daily, take special vitamins and herbs, and spend a lot of time looking in the mirror. They make everyone around them feel inferior or guilty. Superficially, they appear to be perfect stewards of their bodies.

But a good steward is never *so* fixated on taking care of the valued goods that he or she never allows anyone to enjoy them. No temple will last forever, whether in Jerusalem, Angor Wat, or Rome. One ought to worship the God within the temple, not worship the temple itself. The latter is a form of idolatry. A beautiful but impenetrable cathedral is not a temple. One can make one's body into a mausoleum in which the Spirit has succumbed to the noxious fumes of the agents one has used for "buffing." Despite beautiful appearances, the Spirit inside is dead. Gifts are meant to be used and shared. One should not spend so much time at the health club toning one's muscles that one never has time to play baseball with one's children.

Neglect

At the other extreme, too many people neglect their bodies. They pay no attention to their blood pressure or cholesterol. They never exercise or watch their diets. They never get flu shots or mammograms or checkups.

Sometimes people fall into the trap of thinking that caring for themselves in a balanced and healthy way is vanity or selfishness. But such persons may be failing to care for themselves out of a false sense of humility. This is not responsible stewardship, either. The human body is truly a great gift. One *does* need to take good care of one's body. One is duty bound not to neglect it.

Sometimes this sort of attitude is fed by the misinterpretation of the Pauline epistles that I discussed above. Christians, Catholic and otherwise, sometimes neglect their bodies because they think that St. Paul teaches that we should "hate our bodies," as mentioned earlier. But St. Paul did not hate himself. He did not neglect his health. He went to see doctors. He was careful about what he ate. What St. Paul means is that we should not be prodigal with our bodies. Physical pleasure is not evil, but part of the goodness of how God created us.

What St. Paul really means is that we should not be overcome by lust or gluttony, living lives obsessed by the pursuit of pleasure. Nor should we make our bodies into false idols. And, above all, we should not neglect our bodies.

Abuse

Nor should people abuse their own bodies or other people's bodies. It does not matter whether all involved parties have given their rational, autonomous consent to a certain activity. The body is a gift. One is not free to do with it as one would wish. In fact, as St. Paul says, in stunning contrast to the mores of the contemporary world, "you are not your own" (1 Cor 6:19). The steward does not own the property. The rector does not own the cathedral. There is no right to vandalize any human body.

What constitutes vandalism of the body? I suppose customs differ widely from culture to culture. The willful use of dangerous and addictive drugs in ways that are not socially sanctioned (and kept within socially controlled limits) and can cause physical or mental harm will always be one way to vandalize the temple of the Holy Spirit. But tattoos? Body piercing? The elongation of one's earlobes? These practices will legitimately vary, within reason, from place to place and time to time, but within a given culture, there will be excesses that surely constitute vandalism rather than enhancement. There is a difference between art and graffiti.

Among Catholics in particular, however, one sometimes encounters a form of bodily abuse that can falsely mask itself as genuine piety. People sometimes refuse to avoid serious but preventable physical pain and suffering—or even deliberately seek serious physical pain and suffering—for the sake of alleged spiritual gains. For instance, some sincere Catholics will refuse morphine if they have cancer pain, proposing that they have a duty to feel this pain and to unite their sufferings to those of Christ.

This is not good stewardship. Such attitudes may have been fed by the persistence of strains of Jansenism and other heresies that, centuries after having been suppressed, have continued to exert influence on the faithful.[5] Such practices are inconsistent with good stewardship, just as it would be inconsistent for the rector of a cathedral deliberately to destroy the mellifluous sounding bell in the tower of a cathedral for fear that its beautiful sounds would distract people from worship.

Acts of self-denial and penance have their place in the spiritual life. But such gestures are only appropriate if performed within the bounds of moderation and done for one of two legitimate spiritual purposes.

First, such acts can be purely symbolic. As such, they symbolize the finitude of the body and the radical dependence of all human beings on the source of all life and all strength, the one, holy, all-powerful, ever-living, and ever-true God. Performed in a genuinely Christian and spiritual manner, these are small gestures and can have enormous spiritual meaning. Abstaining from certain desired foods or activities that are otherwise legitimate in themselves (for example, meat) would fall into this category. The practice of kneeling when praying would be another.

Second, such acts of self-denial and penance can be acts of discipline or spiritual training. Conscious of the finitude of the human person in the moral, intellectual, and bodily dimensions, one sometimes needs to remind oneself of that finitude in a modest physical way. In part, this reminder helps to prepare one for future suffering that will be occasioned by more serious deprivations. Short periods of fasting, for instance, fall into this category. On occasion, it is good to feel hunger in solidarity with those around the world who are truly starving and to remember that one's own body will likely experience more serious deprivations in the future. Nevertheless, orthodox Christian teaching would not encourage excess in these practices.

Suffering is inevitable in human life. There are times when Christianity teaches that one must accept suffering as the key to accepting the truth of one's humanity, in all its finitude and dignity. This key opens the door to eternal life. This key has the shape of the cross.

But one ought not to seek such suffering for its own sake. Rather, one must accept suffering only when the choice one faces is either to flee from the fullness of life because it will entail suffering or to embrace life and the suffering life entails, to flee from love because it will entail suffering or to embrace love and the suffering love entails. Thus, in the shadow of the cross, the night before he died, Jesus asked the Father to take away the cup of his suffering. Jesus sought to *avoid* the suffering of his impending Passion. And hanging on the cross, Jesus accepted the gall that was the morphine of his day. But Jesus gave himself over to that suffering precisely because without it, God could not have shown human beings the love that redeems them and the life that is promised them. It was this suffering that Jesus could not flee. And this is the only suffering to which Christians are called: the inescapable suffering that is sometimes required in order to affirm life and love. This is the only suffering one can truly unite with the suffering of Christ—that which cannot be avoided if one is to live the Gospel. The altar on which such suffering takes place is the holy of holies, the inner sanctum, the temple of the human body. There the Spirit truly dwells.

Conclusion

Christians have a duty to care for their bodies. Human bodies, in themselves, are good; they are gifts from Almighty God. One only deviates from respect for the goodness of one's body if one is prodigal, neglectful, or abusive of one's own flesh.

Fortunately, because the body is exceptionally well made, caring appropriately for it is generally very easy. Most adult human beings learned the basics of bodily stewardship as children. Good health care professionals really do not need to suggest much more. Eat your vegetables. Do not smoke. Exercise. Do not have sex outside of marriage. If you drink, do so only in moderation. Do not use illicit drugs. Take your medicine.

Despite the problems with managed care and the disgraceful lack of insurance for so many of the poor in this nation, most Americans have much better medical care than almost all other people in the world. One only has to avail oneself of the good things that are available. Christians should lead balanced lives. They should be faithful stewards of the wonderful gift of their bodies.

And even if one has *not* been a good steward until now, it is never too late to change. The prodigal son came to his senses. So can any of us who abuse, worship, or neglect our health. One needs a balanced, holistic sense of oneself. One only gives thanks to God, worships God, and shows one's love for the people of God as a creature—fearfully and wonderfully made—of heart, mind, soul, and body.

The Eucharist is a reminder that Christ heals all aspects of the human person—heart, mind, soul, and body. No aspect of the human person is hateful. God made human beings as embodied persons. Human bodies are good. Christians should pray for the grace to be faithful stewards of so great a gift.

Death and the Immanence of Hope

THE words people use have a remarkable way of shaping their attitudes and their actions.[1] As the Psalms say of those who create idols out of wood and bronze, so it is with those who create sentences out of words, "Those who make them are like them" (Ps 115:8). In this spirit, I would like to investigate the meaning of hope in the care of the dying by examining how the word "hope" is used in clinical settings.

A brief review of the titles of some recent medical journal articles will illustrate how pervasive the language of "hopeless illness" has become. The medical literature is replete with such titles as "Optimum Care for Hopelessly Ill Patients: A Report of the Clinical Care Committee of the Massachusetts General Hospital," "Withdrawing Nutrition from Hopelessly Ill Infants," "The Physician's Responsibility towards Hopelessly Ill Patients: A Second Look," "The Care of the Hopelessly Ill: Proposed Clinical Criteria for Assisted Suicide," and "Dutch GP Cleared after Helping to End Man's 'Hopeless Existence.'"[2] The recently described Groningen protocol for the euthanasia of newborn infants requires that "hopeless and unbearable suffering must be present," and because newborns cannot make this judgment, the doctors must be the ones judging that the suffering is hopeless.[3]

Patients use similar language. "Is there any hope, doc? Or am I a goner?" The maintenance of hope has also been a traditional justification for physicians, nurses, and families to conceal from patients the fact that they are terminally ill. In the early nineteenth century, Thomas Percival wrote, "A physician should not be forward to make gloomy prognostications . . . for the physician should be the minister of hope and comfort to the sick."[4]

The living, almost instinctively, urge the critically ill not to give up: "Don't lose hope. You're a fighter." When approached about the question of whether to discontinue a ventilator or other means of life support, family members frequently say, "I couldn't authorize that. I'd be letting down God. It would be like saying I had lost all hope."

Sadly, some patients, also invoking the word "hope," are drawn in the opposite direction. "It's hopeless, doc. It's all over." Or clinicians might say, echoing the titles of the papers cited above, "This case is hopeless. Why are we wasting our time?" Or, borrowing a page from the Groningen protocol, they might say, "When all hope is lost, I see no reason why it wouldn't be morally justified to help someone to die through assisted suicide or euthanasia."

As a house officer, one of my colleagues with a particularly dark sense of humor once placed above the door to the Intensive Care Unit a sign imitating the one that hung above the gates to Dante's *Inferno*:

> *Lasciate ogne speranza*
> *Voi ch'intrate.*
>
> [Abandon all hope
> You who enter here.][5]

Whatever hope is, being deprived of it seems to be a pretty bad thing. Being ill is bad enough. Being *hopelessly* ill is beyond what any human being was meant to endure. The lament of Job echoes down the corridors of time: "My days are swifter than a weaver's shuttle, and come to their end without hope" (Jb 7:6).

Are clinicians right to try to keep patients from losing hope? Or should they be more realistic and not deprive their patients of the truth, no matter how hopeless? Just what is hope? Must dying always be a truly hopeless state? Even if a patient's dying sometimes seems hopeless, must it be so?

What Is Hope?

I am not sure that anyone writing of the philosophical moral psychology of hope has ever done better job than Thomas Aquinas. Aquinas identified hope as a very specialized type of desire. He explicated hope as a type of desire characterized by having a specialized kind of object. For Aquinas, the object of hope must be (1) clearly good, (2) apparent in the future, (3) difficult or arduous to attain, and yet (4) regarded as possible to attain.[6] What does this mean?

When Aquinas said that the object of hope must be clearly good, he meant that one only hopes for things that one perceives to be good. One hopes for health and long life, and these are clearly good. Only the mentally ill actually hope for pain or misfortune and even then only because they mistakenly believe these things are good for them. When an object is bad, the usual reaction is fear. One hopes for victory and fears defeat. People hope that they will be virtuous in a coming time of trial, yet fear that they might turn out to be weaker than they imagined themselves to be. One hopes for life and fears death. The object of hope is always a perceived good.

Aquinas also noted that hope is always a desire for a future good. One cannot hope for what has already happened. One does not hope for a cure if one is already cured.

Furthermore, hope is a desire for what comes about only arduously or with a very uncertain likelihood. One does not typically need to express deep hope that the sun will rise tomorrow. One says, "I hope my car will start" only if one has some suspicion that it might not start or that it will only start by virtue of some combination of effort and good fortune.

Hope, finally, depends on one's belief that the somewhat uncertain future good that one desires may possibly come to pass. In other words, hope also always depends on an act of faith. Just as one does not say that one hopes for what is absolutely certain, so one does not say that one hopes for what one believes is absolutely impossible. To hope for what one believes to be absolutely impossible is delusional. For example, I genuinely hope that justice and peace can come to pass between the Israeli and the Palestinian peoples. This is a future good that will come to pass, if it all, only with great difficulty. I continue to believe that this can happen, perhaps even before I die. Those who do not believe this can happen might consider me delusional. But I think of it as an expression of legitimate hope. Whatever nurtures the belief that what one desires can actually come to pass nurtures hope.

Hope is thus an interesting emotion. It is a very complex desire, modulated by belief. It is not impulsive desire, but thoughtful desire. It is natural, common, and generally experienced unreflectively. But before proceeding to understand what hope might mean for the dying, it will be necessary next to be clearer about our notions of sickness, death, and dying.

Sickness and Death

Death is an event that strikes us, as human beings, "in our totality."[7] Human death is more than a biological event. Human death is the death of a *person*, as well as an event in nature. Human death is never merely a natural process.[8] A human being dies as a whole person—spirit as well as body.

Bodies decay. They are annihilated. They are broken down and reintroduced into the ecosystem, reconfigured into new bodies, or released as energy into the wide expanse of the cosmos. This happens over and over, and it happens to quarks and stars, viruses and dinosaurs, and paupers and princes. Matter takes on shape in space and time, crumbles, and aggregates again in a new shape elsewhere in space and time.

Persons, however, are unrepeatable events. Each human being is a historical event introduced into the space and time of cosmic and human history. Persons are not recycled.[9] And if that is the case, then the wonder of human birth and the finality of human death are the fundamental human mysteries with which one must grapple. Barring mental incapacity, both birth and death are experiences of which all human beings are aware and that all human beings understand with absolute certitude, without recourse to any religious creed or meditative practice. If persons are not recycled into other persons or other species, then the death of any person can only mean one of two things—utter annihilation or perduring personal existence. The *matter* of human beings is recycled, but the personhood of human beings either dissipates or continues after death.

Persons are embodied. Christianity utterly rejects the notion that human beings are really spirits accidentally taking up residence in bodies. This sort of Gnostic dualism cannot take the events of incarnation, passion, and resurrection seriously because it does not take the reality of human persons seriously. Human beings are matter and mind, blood and water, flesh and spirit. The death of the human person takes place under this same dual aspect. Yet the death of the body and the death of the person are *one* death. Death is not the liberation of the "true self" from the prison of embodied existence. Human death is an event of nature and spirit at once.

Human death is therefore a paradox. The nature of human beings, as embodied creatures, is finite. Death and limitation are the signs of creaturehood. There is only one uncreated and absolute infinity. Only God is infinite. Everything created, by virtue of being created, must be utterly other than God and therefore utterly finite.

Yet as persons, created in the image and likeness of the creator, endowed with intellect, passion, and freedom, each human being is essentially oriented toward the wideness of the cosmos. A person (a being that is, by its nature, a thinking, feeling, and freely willing entity) is essentially an openness to the entire universe of relationships: to other people, to the universe, and, ultimately, to God.[10]

Considering the dual aspects of the human is not the same as dualism. To understand that there are two aspects to the question, what is a human being? is not to say that there are two distinct substances that are somehow linked to each other to make a human being. Persons are not ghosts accidentally inhabiting bodies. Persons live embodied lives but are aware that they are more than mere matter.

And the paradox, then, is this. Our death as embodied, natural, and finite biological beings is absolutely finite, absolutely inevitable, and absolutely passive. Death, in its biological aspect, happens to us. We cannot control it. We cannot avoid it. And it could not be otherwise, for we are creatures.

But at the same time, human death is an experience of *persons*. Human death is not the death of a sparrow. Death is something persons can engage as intelligent, passionate, and free beings oriented always toward a relationship with the transcendent. Death is something we, as persons, enact. As Catholic theologian Karl Rahner wrote, a person's "free, personal, self-affirmation and self-realization achieves in death an absolute determination."[11]

Human death is thus a submission and an achievement at once. We undergo death in its biological aspect. We enact death in its personal aspect. Death in its biological aspect is annihilation. Death in its personal aspect holds forth the possibility that it might be one's ultimate personal act: what one brings actively to death's passive inevitability is the historical disposition of the freedom one has lived over an entire personal lifetime.

Death in Life

It is often said, especially among palliative care specialists, that "death is a part of life." Although this is partly true, and might help some persons overcome their fears of talking about death, when examined carefully, the phrase is not very helpful. In a way, the words can actually sound trite because they reveal only a tiny fraction of the truth. Death is not merely the part of life that comes at the end. Death is an essential aspect of every moment of life. Human beings are conscious of their finitude, conscious of their eventual death. Turtles are not. Yet human beings are also absolutely oriented beyond the horizon of their finitude and death by virtue of their intellect, imagination, feelings, desires, and freedom of will. Humans are beings in essential relationship with the infinity that surrounds them, drawn to that infinity, and conscious always of their own finitude. Death is, almost by nature, present throughout the whole of a human life. Each human being is engaged in the ultimate drama—enacting his or her own death, as his or her own consummation, through the deeds of life, while at the same time conscious of death's inevitability and his or her own powerlessness before death's face.[12] Death is not a simple momentary event at the end of life. It is the summit of the finitude that characterizes every moment in each person's unique human drama.

Death is present in all our human finitude and fallibility. Death is present in our intellectual failures, in our emotional failures, and in our moral failures. But death is especially present in our biological failure. Every drop of blood, every wave of nausea, every creaking joint, and every increase in the prescription for our glasses points ineluctably toward death. As persons we are oriented toward the infinite. As natural creatures we are oriented toward decay. And we know this. No one can deny it.

Death, then, would appear to represent either the pure and perfect distillation or the absolute and irretrievable end of each human person.[13] There is no certain proof which of these is true. But it is the Christian faith that both are true. Death as annihilation came to humankind through Adam's primordial repudiation of God. The death of Jesus, the new Adam, is the ongoing offer to humankind of the absolute perfection of the human person in God. Therefore, death itself, like the life that death actualizes, seems to contain both the possibility of full acceptance and the possibility of full rejection of God.

As in one's living, so in one's dying: one may accept the possibility held out to all persons that death is a redemptive mystery in Christ, or one may reject it. One might, for instance, reject this redemptive offer by affirming only the biological finality of death as annihilation. Consequently, one might live as if death (and therefore life) were ultimately only an utter absurdity. Or one might reject the redemptive mystery by living a life that tries to explain death away—denying the darkness of death and living as if no one ever died, as if death were not genuine biological finality. These are the foundations of hedonism. Or one might reject the redemptive mystery by living a life that treats death (and therefore life) with a sugar-coated dualism—denying the biological meaning of death by triumphally affirming only the spiritual aspect of death. This is what one might call spiritualism.

For the Christian, the death of Christ holds out for humankind the possibility of death as the consummation of a life open to the grace of God. Christ, obedient unto death, affirms both the finality of death as a biological event and the ultimate redemption of the human as personal being oriented to the infinite. To die in Christ is to die in complete and utter openness to the created world and to the creator of the world. To die in Christ is to die open to the Word of God, open to the grace of God. Through the Incarnation of Christ, God becomes transparent to the world and to the human. Through the death of Christ, the human becomes completely transparent to the world and to God. The Christian understands this as a permanent ontological transformation of history. Human death in Christ is no more and no less than this—the very possibility of ultimate human integration.

Hope as a Transcendent Virtue

Hope, as a human desire, must also have the same dual aspect that characterizes the essence of human beings. Hope, therefore, is both natural and transcendent. To hope to have a sunny day, to pass an examination, or to have one's manuscript published are natural hopes. Each of these events is a future good of uncertain prospect, which one may legitimately believe possible. Good people's lives are full of such hopes.

The sick also have such natural hopes. They naturally hope to recover. They naturally hope to be cured. The objects of these hopes are future goods of uncertain prospect that one may often believe (legitimately) are possible to attain. The natural hopes of the sick have been buoyed up enormously by medical progress. At the dawn of this millennium, the natural hopes of the sick can now legitimately include events that patients and physicians could only dream about in previous millennia—or even previous decades. Many deadly infections, many cancers, and even some metabolic disorders can now be cured. Hundreds of illnesses that were once lethal can now be transformed into chronic conditions. All this is cause for great hope. And the promises of future research hold out even further natural hopes for future generations. But natural hopes should not be exaggerated, nor confused with transcendent hope.[14] The natural hopes of the sick cannot legitimately include a denial of the finitude and biological finality of the death of human beings.

For what can one ultimately hope? One cannot avoid death. To deny death by a life of hedonism, seeking only the pleasures of this life, fleeing from the death that is present in every moment of life—in biological, intellectual, emotional, and moral finitude—is to live a life of delusion. To deny death by living in an otherworldly, sugar-coated piety in which everything is spiritualized as if the here-and-now, actual, day-in and day-out struggles and realities of life were not real is to live a life of pitiable fancy. To affirm the awful truth of the finitude of the human and also deny that death might hold the possibility of ultimate, infinite integration is to live a life of ultimate despair.

Is there, then, any hope for the human race? One can only legitimately hope for future desired goods that one considers possible. Human beings, in their personhood, are oriented toward the embrace of the infinite. To have this desire and yet to believe that this desire could never possibly be fulfilled would constitute a form of radical despair about the meaning of the human person in life as well as in death. One could only escape from such despair by trying to suppress one's desire for the infinite, one's quest to know the infinite, and the orientation of one's own human freedom toward the infinite. But this would seem to be the denial of one's personhood—seeking solace from the awful reality of one's belief in the ultimate absurdity of human life by trying to make oneself something less than human.

Centuries ago Thomas Aquinas recognized this critical aspect of human beings—that human beings are essentially oriented toward an end that they cannot achieve by themselves.[15] From a more contemporary psychospiritual perspective, Sebastian Moore has noted how deeply this orientation is ingrained in the human psyche. He understands the quest for meaning as the question, "Am *I* meaningful?" He has noted that all human beings ask this question and cannot answer it themselves. It is a question put always to an unknown other, who must recognize the one who asks it and find him or her to be meaningful. Ultimately, it is a question of whether there is any Other who finds us valuable. At the limit, Moore has argued, it is a question about the existence of a loving God:

> We are much more emotionally involved with God, or at least the question of God, than we like to think or admit. This emotional involvement with God is the key to our self-understanding and to the understanding of religion. It is pre-religious. Religion is the believed-in answer of the unknown other, to the question: "Am I valuable in your eyes?" Unless we can come to understand the question as our question and the most human thing about us, we shall never understand the religious answer as the fulfillment of our whole desire for meaning.[16]

Aquinas recognized that this hope is not simply an emotion, but a habitual predisposition of human persons—a virtue. He recognized that there could only be ultimate hope if there were some possibility that the ultimate desire of human beings might be realized. A just creator, Aquinas reasoned, would need to supply human beings with the possibility of realizing such intelligent desire. He thus distinguished between the universally human moral and intellectual virtues, or the cardinal virtues, and what he called the theological virtues.[17] These virtues would need to be supplied by God's free gift because they were beyond the possibility of human nature alone. God created human beings with an orientation that transcended the finitude of their creatureliness and therefore, if just, would need to supply a transcendent means if their deepest desires were to be fulfilled. The "natural" virtues of prudence, temperance, fortitude, and justice would not suffice. As Aquinas wrote, "The power of principles naturally within us does not extend beyond the capacity of nature. Consequently, in relation to a supernatural end, man needs to be perfected by other principles in addition to these."[18] Because they concern what lies beyond the limits of natural human potential, I prefer to call these the transcendent virtues. These transcendent virtues are the famous trio: faith, hope, and love.

Faith and hope are transcendent in the sense that they concern the limits of human being—the horizon of human experience. As a transcendent virtue, faith concerns what cannot be empirically proved—the limitless realm of knowability that lies beyond the horizon of the merely concrete and the biologically sensible. As a transcendent virtue, hope concerns humankind's unfathomable desire for what lies beyond the human, what human beings cannot humanly give each other or attain on their own.[19]

Just as natural faith in the possible realization of its object is necessary for natural hope, so transcendent faith is also a prerequisite for transcendent hope. As it is written in Hebrews 11:1, "Faith is the assurance [in the King James version, "substance"] of things hoped for." Without faith, there can be no hope.

Faith is also a prerequisite for love. One cannot desire, choose, or trust what one does not believe to exist.[20] One does not love (and cannot be loved by) fantasies.

And ultimately, as Thomas Merton wrote, "All desires but one can fail."[21] The most fundamental of all human desires is the desire to be loved absolutely and unconditionally. This desire expresses Sebastian Moore's fundamental question, "Am I meaningful?" This desire cannot be fulfilled by any human being. No matter how close a couple, how close a family, or how close a friendship, the love all persons seek is a love that is not humanly possible. What human beings seek is beyond the horizon of natural human capacity and experience. What human beings seek is truly transcendent—a possibility only realizable in God. It is a possibility for which one may hope in faith. Its realization depends on one's faith and one's ability to accept the gift that is sought.

Dying in Christian Hope

For what, then, can the dying hope? Certainly they cannot hope for corporeal immortality. And anyone who demands this of God is guilty of pride, trying to be something more than human. Just as certainly, the dying cannot hope for perfect medicine. No matter how sophisticated and successful medical science becomes, no matter what new cures await the biomedical world, and no matter what life-sustaining technologies doctors and nurses may apply, medicine will, with all the natural necessity one can ever know, face its limitations, finitude, and failure. Ultimately, medicine must confront the ineluctable mortality of the creatures to whom it ministers.

Just as certainly, the dying cannot hope to avoid all suffering. Even if all pain were one day perfectly controllable, the experiences of finitude, failure, and loss that are essential to the human condition will always arise as occasions of human suffering on planes far deeper than the suffering brought forth by pain.

Only ultimate meaning can be the proper object of ultimate hope. For the Christian this meaning is disclosed in the form of a person—Jesus Christ. Like St. Paul, Christians can put their trust only in "Christ Jesus our hope" (1 Tim 1:1). Christians must stand before the world, like Peter, proclaiming their "hope in the resurrection of the dead" (Acts 23:6). Christians, believing in God and trusting in God's Word, can share in the death of Jesus—accepting the finality of its natural aspect and engaging the eternity of its personal aspect. Christians look to the resurrection. And resurrection is not resuscitation.[22]

The Christian hope of the dying is the only hope that can transcend death—hope in the love of God. This hope is possible for those who engage death, as they engage life, open to other persons, to the universe, and to God. And God's love, poured out for each individual person, and for everyone else, filling the entire universe in all its parts (Eph 1:23), is enough for us. As Merton wrote, "We can either love God because we hope for something from Him, or we can hope in Him knowing that he loves us. Sometimes we begin with the first, and grow into the second."[23]

As in any other relationship of love, spiritual growth often happens this way. Human beings sometimes start by looking for what they can "get" out of the relationship, but as they fall more and more deeply in love, they grow satisfied with love alone. They grow satisfied with love because they understand it through experience. Similarly, a patient might start out hoping to be cured of cancer or of AIDS, and God may be present in many small and incomplete acts of physical healing along a patient's journey with illness. But it cannot end there. The experience of God's love in this life must finally give a reason for the hope that will even transcend death.

This is our ultimate desire and ultimate fulfillment. God's love is eternal. It is the absolute horizon toward which our personhood irrevocably points. As Merton wrote, "If we place our last hope in something limited, we withdraw our hearts entirely from the service of the living

God. If we continue to love Him as our end, but place our hope in something else together with Him, our love and our hope are not what they should be, for no man can serve two masters."[24]

Let the dying, then, pray with the psalmist, and the living with them, "And now, O Lord, what future do I have? You are my only hope" (Ps 39:8). Our hope is in God's love for us: the wild, free, exuberant, unimaginable expansiveness of God's love for us. Our hope must finally rest in God.

I do not wish to suggest that this is as easy to do as it is to say. Merton again, in his *No Man Is an Island*, wrote, "Only the man who has had to face despair is really convinced that he needs mercy. Those who do not want mercy never seek it. It is better to find God on the threshold of despair than to risk our lives in a complacency that has never felt the need of forgiveness."[25]

Although true of all persons, Merton's observation is often true of the dying. Imminent death brings all the great questions into such clear focus. Out of a confrontation with the possibility of radical despair, the possibility that death means both the annihilation of the body and the annihilation of the person, and the possibility that a life might culminate in a death in which one utterly repudiates the love God offers, someone's ultimate yes to God and final hope in God's love might emerge. Unless one is prepared to consider the possibility that there is no God, one's faith might be merely a reflexive and superficial response to social conditioning. The demon of doubt, as T. S Eliot once said, is inseparable from the spirit of faith.[26]

Hope, therefore, as Merton suggested, is profoundly connected with reconciliation. Ultimate hope is in a transcendent relationship, and that relationship is set right through contrition and forgiveness. This reconciliation, this restoration of right relationship, can happen to any of us, in any of the dying moments of our living, wherein we recognize, on the brink of despair, our own unworthiness and need for God's healing and forgiving love. T. S. Eliot captured this sense of a spiritual quest verging on the brink of despair in the opening lines of his great poem of conversion, "Ash Wednesday":

> Because I do not hope to turn again
> Because I do not hope
> Because I do not hope to turn—[27]

The choice between hope and despair is the radical situation of the dying person. One can emerge from the brink of despair to engage death in hope—desiring nothing but the love of God in death and in every dying moment of one's life. To engage death in such hope requires faith—trust that one's ultimate desire to be loved totally and unconditionally will be fulfilled and that through the death and resurrection of Christ, one's humanity has been made totally transparent to the transcendent. To engage death in faith, hope, and love is to experience the love of God in each dying moment of one's living, reaching its summit in one's corporeal dissolution into the very mystery of God.

This death is the death of baptism. Those who were baptized into the death of Christ believe that they will also rise with him (Rom 6:3–5), believing that the ultimate meaning of personhood arises from the love of God and finds its completion in the love of God. As Eliot wrote, this is "no occupation either, but something given / And taken, in a lifetime's death in love."[28]

This is our hope. No other hope will ultimately sustain us—in life or in death. To despair of such hope is ultimately to despair of the meaningfulness of human life. Christians must therefore "always be ready to give an explanation to anyone who asks [us] for a reason for [our] hope" (1 Pt 3:15).

Implications for Health Care

What might this spirituality mean for those of us who care for the dying? It means, first and foremost, as pointed out by Vaclav Havel, that hope has nothing whatsoever to do with prognosis. It has everything to do with the human spirit. He wrote, "The kind of hope I often think about (especially in situations that are particularly hopeless, such as prison) I understand above all as a state of mind, not a state of the world. Either we have hope within us or we don't; it is a dimension of the soul, and it's not essentially dependent on some particular observation of the world or estimate of the situation. Hope is not prognostication."[29]

This means, of course, that no patient's situation is ever truly hopeless. To speak in such terms narrows the field of human experience to the merely biological and ignores the personal aspects of the patient's dying. If the situation of the dying is truly hopeless, then the situation of the living is also hopeless, for we are all, every one of us, dying in every moment of our living.

I think it also means that clinicians must be careful never to give false hopes to their patients. Puffed up with pride in their scientific achievements, they often promise more natural hope than is realistic. Perhaps it is because their own faith is too weak to sustain their own transcendent hope, let alone that of their patients. So they substitute natural hope in their own technological prowess for transcendent hope in the love of God.

Health care professionals often place their hopes in the wrong place—in the limited and the transitory. Physicians, nurses, respiratory technologists, and other health care professionals should recall the words of T. S. Eliot for their own work as well as for their patients:

I said to my soul, be still, and wait without hope
For hope would be hope for the wrong thing; wait without love
For love would be love of the wrong thing; there is yet faith
But the faith and the hope and the love are all in the waiting.[30]

Hope requires imagination. Health care professionals can help patients to hope if they can teach them to imagine the real.[31] Patients on the brink of despair sometimes only need help imagining that their deepest and absolutely ultimate desires can be fulfilled. Hope requires faith, and faith requires imagination: imagination not as fantasy but as the apprehension of the not yet realized real.

Health care professionals also need to remember that hope is sustained and nurtured in relationship and in community. The ultimate end of human hope is a loving relationship with God. But patients can catch glimpses of that ultimate relationship if health care professionals provide them with evidence that they are still very much a part of the human community.[32] People often build walls around the sick. They project onto the sick their own lack of faith, lack of hope, and lack of love. People can deny their own death by portraying dying persons as essentially different from them.[33] But the dying are part of the living. We bear the death of the Lord deep in our hearts. And the Lord has already borne in himself all our dyings. We need to reassure the dying, even as the bonds of corporeal reality that link them and us together are slowly dissolving, that they are first and foremost persons, and we need to remind them of our faith that their personhood will abide with us now and forever.

Hope is the healing of the dying. When the chemotherapy no longer works, and the radiation dosage limits have been reached, and the pain persists as a gnawing dull reminder of the finitude that is our common lot, the dying, in virtue of their hope, can engage death as their own. "The image of death as passivity and helplessness may well be the greatest American fear."[34] In its material aspect, this passivity is the truth. Not one of us can escape. Death will *happen* to each of us in its biological aspect. But the hope of the dying is not to be found in biology textbooks. For the Christian, death becomes an active process. We actively place our hope in Christ. Our hope is in God's promise of love, which is the only certain hope. Death can be engaged in its personal aspect by those who submit to its biological finality and yet at one and the same time find in death the absolute consummation and fulfillment of a life lived in "a living hope, through the resurrection of Jesus Christ from the dead" (1 Pt 1:3). This sort of transcendent hope can be immanent in the process of dying. "May your kindness, Lord, be upon us; we have put our hope in you" (Ps 33:22).

The Communication of the Dead

THOSE who are most neglected by our current health care system are perhaps those who are left behind after a patient dies. Although no firm data exist, in an era in which most persons in developed nations live in large cities and suburbs rather than small, close-knit communities, it seems that it is rare for a physician or nurse to attend a patient's wake or funeral.[1] One observer has noted that we now practice "stranger medicine" in the United States—patients and their health care professionals have generally never met before the episode of care at hand.[2] This is true even of the care of the dying. Patients often come to the hospital to die, cared for by people who have never met them before. Yet if "stranger medicine" describes the relationship between health care professionals and patients, it may be too meek a term to describe the relationship between health care professionals and the bereaved. This relationship may more aptly be called "alien medicine." The family and friends of dying patients often never get to know their loved ones' doctors and nurses, and doctors and nurses rarely ever get to know them. And even when health care professionals have come to know them, making their acquaintances as they accompany the patient through life's final journey, the death of the patient usually marks the end of any relationship with family or friends. The loved ones, who might have been "resident aliens" in the hospital for a brief period of time, are quickly "deported." Once the body leaves the floor, these loved ones are never seen or heard from again.

Some of this is changing. Certainly "alien medicine" has never been the practice of hospice workers, who pay close attention to the care of the family both before and after the patient's death. Newly created programs of palliative care are beginning to stress the importance of caring for the bereaved as well.

But how does one care for the bereaved? Beyond a stiff and perfunctory expression of condolences at the loss of the patient, what can a clinician say to those who mourn? Is there a spirituality of mourning about which physicians, nurses, social workers, and other health care professionals can learn?

Much could be said about this subject—too much for one chapter in a book. I make no pretense of trying to give a crash course in bereavement therapy or attending to the spiritual needs of those who have lost loved ones. Others have done this much better than I.[3] What I hope to do in this chapter, however, is to explore one important question in the spirituality of bereavement: the question of whether and how one can pray to the dead. The reader may have had more personal than professional experience with this question, but that may only mean that the line of demarcation between the personal and the professional has been drawn in the wrong place. I am sure that the family and friends of many patients have asked this question after their loved one has died. A professional ought to be prepared to grapple with it.

Catholic theology has long held a robust notion of the communion of saints—a community that includes both the living and the dead. Given a traditional belief in purgatory, almost all believing Catholics will also accept that one can pray *for* the dead. But it is another question altogether to ask whether one can one pray *to* the dead. T. S. Eliot, in describing a profound episode of prayer, drew a fundamental link between spiritual experience and conversation with the dead.

> If you came this way,
> Taking the route you would be likely to take
> From the place you would be likely to come from,
> . . . .
> It would be the same at the end of the journey,
> If you came at night like a broken king,
> If you came by day not knowing what you came for,
> It would be the same, when you leave the rough road
> And turn behind the pig-sty to the dull façade
> And the tombstone. And what you thought you came for
> Is only a shell, a husk of meaning
> From which the purpose breaks only when it is fulfilled

If at all. Either you had no purpose
Or the purpose is beyond the end you figured
And is altered in fulfillment. There are other places
Which are also the world's end, some at the sea jaws,
Or over a dark lake, in a desert or a city—
But this is the nearest, in place and time,
Now and in England.
                    If you came this way,
Taking any route, starting from anywhere,
At any time or at any season,
It would always be the same: you would have to put off
Sense and notion. You are not here to verify,
Instruct yourself, or inform curiosity
Or carry report. You are here to kneel
Where prayer has been valid. And prayer is more
Than an order of words, the conscious occupation
Of the praying mind, or the sound of the voice praying.
And what the dead had no speech for, when living,
They can tell you, being dead: the communication
Of the dead is tongued with fire beyond the language of the living.
Here, the intersection of the timeless moment
Is England and nowhere. Never and always.[4]

Eliot, it seems, believed that one can pray to the dead. He believed there is a communication between souls on both sides of the grave that is so profound it cannot be captured by words. But what could this mean for those who have just lost a husband or a wife or a child or a parent or a very dear friend? Can one help a bereaved person to pray to the loved one he or she has lost? Can a nurse or a physician communicate with a dead patient, or would this be the height of blasphemy in the cool, scientific world of contemporary medicine?

I cannot answer all these questions. But I can offer a few simple thoughts. First, praying to the dead has nothing to do with the world of the occult. I am continually frustrated by the popularity of television shows that purport to put people in contact with the dead through various kinds of conjuring. This sort of spectacle is both a fictional exploitation of the dead and a manipulative exploitation of those who mourn them. We do not conjure the dead. Every honest wife should know that she will have no more control over her husband once he is dead than she had while he was living! Sorcery is not genuine spirituality.

One ought never attempt to manipulate God or to manipulate those whose lives are now "hidden with Christ in God" (Col 3:3).

Second, I *do* believe that the dead are with us in memory. If the dead communicate with us only through memory, however, then that communication is not a genuine conversation. The memories we have of the dead are often beautiful and good. In surging waves, at a moment's notice, and with or without provocation, memories come flooding into the lives of those who have recently lost loved ones. An old photo, a necktie, or a piece of jewelry can evoke all the meanings with which that item had been invested but had never been noticed or verbalized in life. The smell of a closet can move one far beyond its confines. A few notes of a favorite melody can almost seem to bring the one we loved before us, humming. We connect these present events to past events—events warm in the memory. They can bring a smile, a tear, or both. But such experiences are not prayers to the dead. They are not, in themselves, instances in which one would really be talking to the dead or in which the dead would really be talking to the living.

Memories fade. It is a central Christian belief that people do not. We remember the names of only a small number of extremely famous people who lived long ago—Moses, Plato, the Buddha, Mohammed, St. Francis. Those whose fame lasts more than a few decades are but the tiniest fraction of 1 percent of all the persons who have ever lived. Few people can even remember the maiden name of their own great-grandmother. One's own memories cannot last more than a lifetime. Memories are good, but memories do not constitute true conversation with an immortal soul.

Third, some persons are tempted to believe that the dead live on only through their deeds, through the fruit of the good works one can attribute to them long after they are gone. For example, a man might dig an excellent water well that benefits thousands of people over hundreds of years. Or a woman might work extremely hard at a job, saving the income to pay tuition for a child whose career successes continue long after she is gone. Or someone might plant a garden that continues to grow, flourish, and give delight for successive generations.

These are all good things for which we should truly be grateful to the dead. But one cannot pray to a consequence. Temporal consequences do not participate in any eternal, transcendent reality. Eventually, all gardens fade. Eventually, every well runs dry. No human deed is eternal. If I am to be present to those who follow me, my deeds will not be enough for them. The bereaved person cannot hope to pray to the abstraction of the ongoing good deeds of a loved one. That would not be a conversation with a person, nor would it be eternal.

Yet I do believe that there is a way in which the dead are still with us and that we can pray *to* them and not just *for* them. This way is not through the occult, nor is it merely an experience resident in the memory or the conscious recognition of their abstract presence to us as the agents who effected good deeds that continue to bear fruit. I believe the dead are really with us—as persons. This way is called, in Catholic theology, the communion of saints.

Prayer and of the Communion of Saints

A fellow Franciscan friar once told me a story about his conversation with a woman who had recently lost a very dear friend. Her friend had helped this woman and her family enormously after her husband had become quadriplegic in an accident. His assistance to this woman, her husband, and their young son, always given with good cheer, had never faded over more than a decade. He had become a part of the family.

But her friend had died suddenly and prematurely. And complicating her grief was the exposure of a secret about her friend that was widely circulated posthumously and without his prior authorization. The woman had become furious—almost uncontrollably angry—not at those who had exposed the secret but at her recently deceased friend. She said to the friar counseling her, "I never knew this about him. Why didn't he tell me? We were so close that he was like a brother and a father and a son all rolled into one for us. I'm so angry. Why didn't he tell me?"

The wise friar saw that it would do no good to explain to her how this had happened, to inform her of the fact that most people keep many things secret in life, or to suggest that her reaction might be a form of psychological projection. He was wise enough to avoid all of that. She was inconsolably angry. He knew of no rational arguments or insights that would change her. And so he said, "Gosh, I don't know why he never told you, Catherine. Why don't you just go home and ask him? I'm sure he can explain why better than I can." Immediately she began to weep.

"Why don't you just go home and ask him?" This simple sentence expresses profound belief in the communion of saints—the belief that the dead are still with us and that we can commune with them. "And what the dead had no speech for, when living, they can tell you, being dead": That is the kind of real relationship with the dead that I believe is possible.

But how is this so? Margaret Atwood, in her poem "Variations on the Word *Sleep*," suggested a way that this might be so. Atwood wrote of a woman's feelings toward her husband. She did not set out in the poem to explain how the dead might still be with us. But she explained how those who have loved us remain with us. They are not just memories or abstract ongoing consequences. She wrote,

> I would like to be the air
> that inhabits you for a moment
> only. I would like to be that unnoticed
> & that necessary.[5]

The relevance to the issue at hand is this: all those who have ever loved us inhabit us deeply, now. They are inside us, like the air we breathe. Like the God to whom they have gone, the God who St. Augustine told us is "nearer to us than we are to ourselves," the dead are with us.[6] We may never have noticed, but they have become a necessary part of who we are. They really are that close—close enough to talk to. They are part of what constitutes us as persons.

Gerard Manley Hopkins had a similar insight in his poem "The Blessed Virgin Compared to the Air We Breathe." He understood this very personal and intimate metaphor at a profound spiritual level. He wrote,

> This air, which, by life's law,
> My lung must draw and draw
> Now but to breathe its praise,
> Minds me in many ways
> Of her who not only
> Gave God's infinity
> Dwindled to infancy
> Welcome in womb and breast,
> Birth, milk, and all the rest

But mothers each new grace
That does now reach our race

. . . .
        I say that we are wound
With mercy round and round
As if with air: the same
Is Mary, more by name.

. . . .
And men are meant to share
Her life as life does air.[7]

Our finitude has both an outer and an inner horizon. There is a limit to how far we can see out over the ocean and a limit to how far we can see peering down into its depths. We can extend ourselves further, or we can search more deeply within ourselves, but there is a beyond to both dimensions. The Christian faith is that love is what lies beyond both the horizon before us and the horizon within us.

The people who have loved us deeply, even though they have died, have fallen into the mystery of the God—the God who is the Love beyond all human love and the Beyond of all the horizons that circumscribe our lives. This God, as St. Bonaventure once wrote, is the one "whose center is everywhere and whose circumference is nowhere."[8] The dead are with us in that Holy Love.

That Love is in England and nowhere. It is at the university medical center and at St. Elsewhere's. It is everywhere and nowhere. And if those who mourn the dead would but listen, they could hear their dearly departed tell them of that Love. Love's language looms long beyond the lamentations of the living.

Postscript

A Residency Graduation Prayer
(St. Vincent's Hospital–Manhattan)

All powerful, all holy, all loving
Good and gracious God,

We thank you and we praise you for the privilege of caring for the sick;
For the mysterious beauty of the human body which you have created;
For the gifts of the earth by which we heal;
For the power of your presence in our professional lives.

We ask your grace that we may never consider our intelligence to be
    sufficient without fervor;
Knowledge without awe;
Counseling without respect;
Examination without reverence;
Diagnosis without meaning;
Prognosis without hope;
Therapy without compassion.

We pray that we may always be grateful to those who have taught us
    this art.
We pray together for the humility to remain students forever.
We pray today that you will bless our residents as they graduate,
That they may carry within themselves a little bit of this place of heal-
    ing and learning wherever their careers may take them,
And that, in the spirit of St. Vincent de Paul, they may always hold a
    special place in their hearts for the sick and the poor of our world.

Amen.

Acknowledgments

Aᴸᴸ scriptural quotes are from the *New Revised Standard Version Bible* (New York: National Council of the Churches of Christ in the United States, 1989). Two chapters are based on work I have published previously. Chapter 3 is based on "Appearance and Morality: Ethics and Otolaryngology—Head and Neck Surgery," *Otolaryngology Head and Neck Surgery* 126 (2002): 4–7, reprinted with the permission of the American Academy of Otolaryngology Head and Neck Surgery, copyrighted © 2002, all rights reserved. Chapter 8 is based on "A Franciscan Spirituality of Health Care," *New Theology Review* 14, no. 4 (2001): 44–50.

Selections from literary works are quoted with the kind permission of the publishers. The excerpt from "Variations on the Word *Sleep*" is from Margaret Atwood, *Selected Poems II: Poems Selected and New, 1976–1986* (Boston: Houghton Mifflin, 1987), copyright © 1987 by Margaret Atwood, reprinted by permission of Houghton Mifflin Company, all rights reserved. The excerpt from "Little Gidding" is from T. S. Eliot, *Four Quartets* (New York: Harcourt, Brace, and World, 1968), reprinted with permission.

Notes

Chapter 1 The Numinous, the Medical, and the Moral

1. The talks from the 2002–3 series and the 2004–5 series have been edited by Alan Astrow and published online in the *Yale Journal for Humanities in Medicine*. These edited talks can be accessed at http://info.med.yale.edu/intmed/hummed/yjhm/spirit2004/spiritintro2004.htm.

2. Albeit coupled with the belief that although natural law ought not contradict revealed religious truth, it is ultimately insufficient for understanding the fullness of moral truth, which does require revelation.

3. Daniel P. Sulmasy, "Every *Ethos* Implies a *Mythos*: Bioethics and Faith," in *Notes from a Narrow Ridge: Religion and Bioethics*, ed. Dena S. Davis and Laurie Zoloth, 227–46 (Frederick, MD: University Publishing Group, 1999).

4. Rudolf Otto, *The Idea of the Holy*, trans. John W. Harvey (London: Oxford University Press, 1957), 5–7.

5. Ibid., 12 ff.

6. Sigmund Freud, *Civilization and Its Discontents*, trans. James Strachey (New York: W. W. Norton, 1961), 11–20.

7. T. S. Eliot, "The Dry Salvages, II," in *Four Quartets* (New York: Harcourt, Brace, and World, 1971), 39.

8. Luigi Giussani, *The Religious Sense*, trans. John Zucchi (Montreal: McGill-Queen's University Press, 1997), 9.

9. Ernest Kurtz and Katherine Ketcham, *The Spirituality of Imperfection* (New York: Bantam, 1992), 140.

10. Francis of Assisi, "Admonition 19," in *Francis of Assisi: Early Documents*, vol. 1, *The Saint*, ed. Regis J. Armstrong, J. A. Wayne Hellman, and William J. Short (New York: New City Press, 1999), 135.

11. Edmund D. Pellegrino and David C. Thomasma, *A Philosophical Basis of Medical Practice: Towards a Philosophy and Ethic of the Healing Professions* (New York: Oxford University Press, 1981), 119–52.

Chapter 2 Letter to a Young Intern

1. Thomas Merton, "Letter to James H. Forrest, Feb. 1, 1961," in *The Hidden Ground of Love: The Letters of Thomas Merton on Religious Experience and*

Social Concern, ed. William H. Shannon, 294–97 (New York: Farrar, Straus and Giroux, 1985).

Chapter 3 Catholic Christianity and the Meaning of Healing

1. See http://www.chausa.org/aboutcha/factsheet.pdf.

2. Niels Bohr, *Atomic Theory and the Description of Nature* (New York: Cambridge University Press, 1961), 18.

3. Bernard J. F. Lonergan, *Insight: A Study of Human Understanding* (San Francisco: Harper and Row, 1958), 245–67.

4. Frank Davidoff, Susan Deutsch, Kathleen Egan, and Jack Ende, *Who Has Seen a Blood Sugar? Reflections on Medical Education* (Philadelphia: American College of Physicians, 1996).

5. Ewert Cousins, trans., *Bonaventure: The Soul's Journey into God, the Tree of Life, the Life of St. Francis* (New York: Paulist Press, 1978), 190.

Chapter 4 Appearance and Morality

1. Albert Borgmann, *Technology and the Character of Contemporary Life* (Chicago: University of Chicago Press, 1984), 81.

2. Ibid., 80.

3. Pellegrino and Thomasma, *Philosophical Basis of Medical Practice*, 207–20.

4. Daniel P. Sulmasy, "What Is an Oath and Why Should a Physician Swear One?" *Theoretical Medicine and Bioethics* 20 (1999): 329–46.

5. S. E. Asch, "Forming Impressions of Personality," *Journal of Abnormal and Social Psychology* 41 (1946): 258–90.

6. Plato, *The Symposium*, trans. Christopher Gill (Harmondsworth, UK: Penguin Classics, 1999), 36–39.

7. Augustine, *City of God*, trans. Henry Bettenson (London: Penguin Classics, 1982), 1074.

8. Plato, *Symposium*, 37.

9. J. M. Weaver and M. B. Flynn, "Hemicorporectomy," *Journal of Surgical Oncology* 73 (2000): 117–24.

10. Plato, *The Republic*, trans. G. M. A. Grube (Indianapolis: Hackett, 1974), 163.

11. Augustine, *City of God*, 850.

12. Alasdair MacIntyre, *Dependent Rational Animals: Why Human Beings Need the Virtues* (Chicago: Open Court, 1999), 100.

13. Ibid., 136.

14. To the best of my knowledge, the only official English version of the biography is in C. C. Martindale, *From Bye-Ways and Hedges* (London: Burns, Oates, and Washbourne, 1935), 3–27. The version told here is adapted from notes taken at a lecture on medicine by the late monsignor Luigi Giussani. I was aided in the translation from the Italian by Elvira Parravicini, M.D.

Chapter 5   The Prodigal Profession

1. Maurice H. Lipper, Bruce J. Hillman, Robert D. Pates, Pippa M. Simpson, Jean M. Mitchell, and D. J. Ballard, "Ownership and Utilization of MR Imagers in the Commonwealth of Virginia," *Radiology* 195 (1995): 217–21.

2. Paul Starr, *The Social Transformation of Medicine* (New York: Basic Books, 1982).

3. Victor G. Freeman, Saif S. Rathore, Kevin P. Weinfurt, Kevin A. Schulman, and Daniel P. Sulmasy, "Lying for Patients: Physician Deception of Third Party Payers," *Archives of Internal Medicine* 159 (1999): 2263–70; Matthew K. Wynia, Deborah S. Cummins, Jonathan B. VanGeest, and Ira B. Wilson, "Physician Manipulation of Reimbursement Rules for Patients: Between a Rock and a Hard Place," *Journal of the American Medical Association* 283 (2000): 1858–65; Rachel M. Werner, Caleb G. Alexander, Angela Fagerlin, and Peter A. Ubel, "The "Hassle Factor": What Motivates Physicians to Manipulate Reimbursement Rules?" *Archives of Internal Medicine* 162 (2002): 1134–39.

4. Dante Alighieri, *Inferno*, trans. Allen Mandelblaum (New York: Bantam, 1986).

Chapter 6   Aesculapion

1. Robert A. Wilcox and Emma M. Whitham, "The Symbol of Modern Medicine: Why One Snake Is More than Two," *Annals of Internal Medicine* 138 (2003): 673–77.

2. The story is difficult to track down. Wilcox and Whitham (above, note 1), tell the story and cite as their source Emma J. Edelstein and Ludwig Edelstein, *Asclepius: Collection and Interpretation of the Testimonies* (Baltimore: Johns Hopkins University Press, 1998). On pages 41–42 the Edelsteins cite a similar story from Ovid that makes no reference to the staff. But they also cite Hyginus, *Astonomica* 2. 14, and this story describes both snake and staff in the healing of Glaucus by Aesculapius, yet they provide no source for the story beyond this Latin text (pp. 367–68). Further complicating matters, they are uncertain about the contribution this story makes to the cult of Aesculapius, citing the idea that the snake sheds its skin as a sign of regeneration associated

symbolically with healing. Still, they are clear that the single snake wrapped around a staff became the symbol of Aesculapius and of the medical profession in the ancient world (pp. 227–31). The most readily available English translation of the story can be found by accessing "Asklepios, in Theoi Project: Guide to Greek Mythology," http://www.theoi.com/Ouranios/Asklepios.html.

3. Edward Tenner, *Why Things Bite Back: Technology and the Revenge of Unintended Consequences* (New York: Alfred A. Knopf, 1996).

4. Inea Bushnaq, ed. and trans., *Arab Folktales* (New York: Pantheon, 1986), 44–45.

5. Daniel P. Sulmasy, "Finitude, Freedom, and Suffering," in *Pain Seeking Understanding: Suffering, Medicine, and Faith*, ed. Mark J. Hanson and Margaret Mohrman, 83–102 (Cleveland: Pilgrim Press, 1999).

6. Joseph Butler, *Five Sermons Preached at the Rolls Chapel and a Dissertation upon the Nature of Virtue* (New York: Bobbs Merrill, 1950), 15.

7. Ernest Kurtz and Katherine Ketcham, *The Spirituality of Imperfection* (New York: Bantam, 1992), 235–36.

Chapter 7 The Man Born Blind

1. References to "the Jews" in this passage (and others in the New Testament, especially the Gospel of John) have unfortunately been misinterpreted and abused at times by so-called Christians in order to justify anti-Semitic attitudes and actions. John's use of "the Jews" probably reflects both Jesus's struggles with the Jewish religious authorities during his lifetime and the struggles of the Jewish Christian community at the time this Gospel was composed, a century later, when the mainstream Jewish community rejected and even persecuted this community. Thus, references to "the Jews" are best interpreted as symbols of all those who reject the message of Jesus and persecute those who believe it. These references ought not to be understood as attacks on the Jewish people. See Sandra M. Schneiders, *Written That You May Believe: Encountering Jesus in the Fourth Gospel* (New York: Crossroads, 1999), 34–35, and Raymond E. Brown, *An Introduction to the Gospel of John* (New York: Doubleday, 2003), 157–75.

2. Sulmasy, "Finitude, Freedom, and Suffering," 83–102.

3. John Hick, *Evil and the God of Love* (London: Macmillan, 1996).

4. Reinhold Niebuhr, *The Nature and Destiny of Man*, vol. 1 (New York: HarperCollins, 1996), 228–31.

Chapter 8 Beatitudes

1. This was one of the central themes of my recent book titled *The Rebirth of the Clinic: An Introduction to Spirituality in Health Care* (Washington, DC: Georgetown University Press, 2006).

2. Daniel P. Sulmasy, M. Gregg Bloche, Jean M. Mitchell, and Jack Hadley, "Physicians' Ethical Views about Cost-Containment Methods," *Archives of Internal Medicine* 160 (2000): 649–57.

3. Jack Hadley, Jean M. Mitchell, Daniel P. Sulmasy, and M. Gregg Bloche, "Financial Incentives, HMO Market Penetration, and Physicians' Practice Styles and Satisfaction," *Health Services Research* 34, no. 1, pt. 2 (1999): 307–21.

4. Mike Norburt, "Primary Care Physicians Caught in Productivity Squeeze," *American Medical News*, September 20, 2004; Julie A. Jacobs, "How Tough Is Life? One State Has the Facts and Figures," *American Medical News*, August 13, 2001.

5. Francis of Assisi, "Admonition 14," in *Francis and Clare: The Complete Works*, trans. Regis J. Armstrong and Ignatius C. Brady (New York: Paulist Press, 1982), 32.

6. Richard Rohr, "Epiphany: You Can't Go Home Again," *St. Anthony Messenger* 108 (January 2001): 12.

7. William Osler, "Aequanimitas," in *Aequanimitas, with Other Addresses to Medical Students, Nurses, and Practitioners of Medicine*, 3rd ed. (New York: McGraw-Hill, 1906), 6.

8. Albert W. Wu, S. Folkman, Stephen J. McPhee, and Bernard Lo, "Do House Officers Learn from Their Mistakes?" *Journal of the American Medical Association* 265 (1991): 2089–94; Albert W. Wu, S. Folkman, Stephen J. McPhee, and Bernard Lo, "How House Officers Cope with Their Mistakes," *Western Journal of Medicine* 159 (1993): 565–69.

9. Francis of Assisi, "Admonition 27," in *Francis and Clare*, 35.

10. Francis of Assisi, "Prayer before the Crucifix," in *Francis of Assisi: Early Documents*, 1:40.

11. T. S. Eliot, "Little Gidding," *Four Quartets* (New York: Harcourt, Brace, World, 1971); cf. Julian of Norwich, *Showings*, trans. Edmund Colledge and James Walsh (New York: Paulist Press, 1978), 225, 248.

12. Francis of Assisi, "Admonition 13," in *Francis and Clare*, 32.

13. Francis of Assisi, "Admonition 15," in *Francis and Clare*, 32.

14. Daniel P. Sulmasy, "Are Health-Plan Incentives Hurting Generalist-Specialist Relationships?" in *Ethical Choices: Case Studies for Medical Practice*, ed. L. Snyder, 163–68 (Philadelphia: American College of Physicians, 2005).

15. Regis J. Armstrong, J. A. Wayne Hellmann, and William J. Short, eds., *Francis of Assisi: Early Documents*, vol. 2, *The Founder* (New York: New City Press, 2000), 89.

Chapter 9 The Blood of Christ

1. Ludwig Wittgenstein, *Tractatus Logico-Philosophicus* (New York: Routledge, 1990), 79. This approach is so novel that I may be the first person

ever to write the names Francis of Assisi and Wittgenstein in a sentence that contains no negations. See also Iris Murdoch, *Metaphysics as a Guide to Morals* (Harmondsworth, UK: Penguin, 1992), 234.

2. Wittgenstein, *Tractatus Logico-Philosophicus*, 187.

3. T. S. Eliot, *The Complete Poems and Plays* (New York: Harcourt, Brace, Jovanovich, 1971), 119.

4. Regis J. Armstrong, J. A. Wayne Hellman, and William J. Short, eds., *Francis of Assisi: Early Documents*, vol. 3, *The Prophet* (New York: New City Press, 2001), 333.

5. Bonaventure. *Collations on the Six Days* (*Collationes in Hexaëmeron*), trans. José deVink (Paterson, NJ: Saint Anthony's Guild, 1970), 179.

6. *Hacceitas* or "thisness" refers to Scotus's view that each existing thing has a particular specification of its universal form or essence by which it exists uniquely as an individual. This view does not go so far as Leibnitz's doctrine of individual essences. See Thomas A. Shannon and Mary Beth Ingham, "The Ethical Method of John Duns Scotus," *Spirit and Life* 3 (1993): 63–65.

7. Cousins, *Bonaventure*, 193–94.

8. Regis J. Armstrong and Ignatius C. Brady, trans. and eds., *Francis and Clare* (New York: Paulist Press, 1982), 37–39.

9. Armstrong, Hellman, and Short, *Francis of Assisi*, 2:243.

10. Armstrong, Hellman, and Short, *Francis of Assisi*, 1:184–85.

11. Cousins, *Bonaventure*, 187.

12. Armstrong, Hellman, and Short, *Francis of Assisi*, 2:293.

13. The language quoted here invokes the marked parallels between Celano's biography of St. Francis and Dylan Thomas's poem, "The Force That through the Green Fuse Drives the Flower," in Dylan Thomas, *The Poems of Dylan Thomas*, ed. David Jones (New York: New Directions, 1971), 77.

14. Cousins, *Bonaventure*, 187.

15. Armstrong, Hellman, and Short, *Francis of Assisi*, 1:124.

16. Cousins, *Bonaventure*, 250.

17. Ibid., 190.

18. Armstrong, Hellman, and Short, *Francis of Assisi*, 2:250.

19. The language here alludes to Dylan Thomas's poem "There Was a Savior," in Thomas, *Poems of Dylan Thomas*, 152–54.

20. Cousins, *Bonaventure*, 305.

21. Ibid.

22. Ibid., 306.

23. Armstrong, Hellman, and Short, *Francis of Assisi*, 1:281.

24. Dante Alighieri, *Paradiso*, ed. and trans. Allen Mandelbaum (Berkeley and Los Angeles: University of California Press, 1982), canto 11, lines 106–8. The translation is mine.

25. Francis Thompson, "Franciscus Christificatus," in *The Francis Book*, ed. Roy Gasnick (New York: Macmillan, 1980), 101.

26. Armstrong, Hellman, and Short, *Francis of Assisi*, 1:274.

27. Ibid., 280.

28. Armstrong, Hellman, and Short, *Francis of Assisi*, 2:2–4.

29. "Cantico delle Creature," trans. Armstrong and Brady, *Francis and Clare*, 39.

30. Armstrong, Hellman, and Short, *Francis of Assisi*, 2:121–23.

31. I am invoking the language of Dylan Thomas's poem "A Refusal to Mourn the Death, by Fire, of a Child in London," *Poems of Dylan Thomas*, 191–92.

32. Cousins, *Bonaventure*, 318.

33. Ibid.

34. Armstrong, Hellman, and Short, *Francis of Assisi*, 1:281.

35. See Paul Ramsey, *The Patient as Person* (New Haven, CT: Yale University Press, 1970); Richard A. McCormick, *How Brave a New World?* (Garden City, NY: Doubleday, 1981), 10–12. McCormick explains the traditional Catholic view that in the Fall of Adam and Eve, human beings lost only the likeness of God, but retained the image of God as the source of their dignity. He distinguishes this from a traditionally Protestant view, as articulated by Karl Barth, that the Fall eliminated both the image and the likeness of God so that human beings derive their dignity solely from God's free gift of grace in the birth, death, and resurrection of Jesus. Barth called this dignity "alien" in the sense that it cannot be claimed to be intrinsic to the fallen nature of human beings. A Catholic is free to believe not only that there is an intrinsic dignity to humanity but also that there is an additional dignity bestowed on us by the saving event of Jesus Christ.

36. Christopher J. Kauffman, *Ministry and Meaning: A Religious History of Catholic Health Care in the United States* (New York: Crossroad, 1995), 132.

37. Armstrong, Hellman, and Short, *Francis of Assisi*, 2:359, 360; Armstrong and Brady, *Francis and Clare*, 220.

38. See the encyclical letter by Pope John Paul II, *Evangelium Vitae*, http://www.vatican.va/edocs/ENG0141/_INDEX.HTM.

39. Cousins, *Bonaventure*, 254.

40. Cf. Thomas, "There Was a Savior," 152–54.

41. Cousins, *Bonaventure*, 191.

42. Thomas, "There Was a Savior," 152–54.

43. Armstrong, Hellman, and Short, *Francis of Assisi*, 1:52, 54, 56, 117, 128–29, 136; Armstrong and Brady, *Francis and Clare*, 64, 67–69, 71.

44. Armstrong, Hellman, and Short, *Francis of Assisi*, 1:540.

Chapter 10 The Temple of the Holy Spirit

1. Mircea Eliade, *The Sacred and the Profane: The Nature of Religion*, trans. Willard R. Trask (New York: Harcourt, Brace, Jovanovich, 1959), 20–29.

2. Augustine, *On Christian Doctrine*, bk. 1, chap. 25, Christian Classics Ethereal Library, Early Church Fathers, v. 2.0, http://www.ccel.org/fathers2/NPNF1-02/npnf1-02-32.htm#P4635_2551579.

3. Ali H. Mokdad, Earl S. Ford, Barbara A. Bowman, William H. Dietz, Frank Vinicor, Virginia S. Bales, and James S. Marks, "Prevalence of Obesity, Diabetes, and Obesity-Related Health Risk Factors, 2001," *Journal of the American Medical Association* 289 (2003): 76–79.

4. Carol A. Ciesielski, "Sexually Transmitted Diseases in Men Who Have Sex with Men: An Epidemiologic Review," *Current Infectious Disease Reports* 5 (2003): 145–52.

5. Jansenism began as a seventeenth-century religious movement in France, holding a doctrine of predestination and encouraging an austere piety and harsh morality. Although condemned as heretical by Pope Innocent X in 1653, it continued to have an influence on Catholicism for centuries, especially in Ireland.

Chapter 11 Death and the Immanence of Hope

1. George Lakoff and Mark Johnson, *Metaphors We Live By* (Chicago: University of Chicago Press, 1980).

2. Clinical Care Committee of the Massachusetts General Hospital, "Optimum Care for Hopelessly Ill Patients: A Report of the Clinical Care Committee of the Massachusetts General Hospital," *New England Journal of Medicine* 295 (1976): 362–64; Jerome L. L'Ecuyer, "Withdrawing Nutrition from Hopelessly Ill Infants," *Journal of Pediatrics* 114 (1989): 339–40; Sidney H. Wanzer, Daniel D. Federman, S. James Adelstein, Christine K. Cassel, Edwin H. Cassem, Ronald E. Cranford, Edward W. Hook, Bernard Lo, Charles G. Moertel, Peter Safar, Alan Stone, and Jan van Eys, "The Physician's Responsibility towards Hopelessly Ill Patients: A Second Look," *New England Journal of Medicine* 320 (1989): 844–49; Timothy E. Quill, Christine K. Cassel, and Diane E. Meier, "The Care of the Hopelessly Ill: Proposed Clinical Criteria for Assisted Suicide," *New England Journal of Medicine* 327 (1992): 1830–34; Tony Sheldon, "Dutch GP Cleared after Helping to End Man's 'Hopeless Existence,'" *British Medical Journal* 321 (2000): 1174.

3. Eduard Verhagen and Pieter J. J. Sauer, "The Groningen Protocol—Euthanasia in Severely Ill Newborns," *New England Journal of Medicine* 352 (2005): 959–62.

4. Thomas Percival, *Percival's Medical Ethics*, ed. C. D. Leake (Huntington, NY: Robert E. Krieger, 1975), 91.

5. Dante Alighieri, *Inferno*, trans. A. Mandelbaum (Berkeley and Los Angeles: University of California Press, 1980), canto 3, line 9.

6. Thomas Aquinas, *Summa Theologiae*, 1-2, q. 40, a. 1, trans. J. P. Reid (New York: McGraw-Hill, 1963).

7. Karl Rahner, *On the Theology of Death*, trans. Charles H. Henkey (New York: Herder and Herder, 1961), 21.

8. Ibid., 46.

9. Reincarnation, a dogma of many Eastern religions, cannot, of course, be empirically proved or disproved, anymore than the Christian faith and its dogmas can be empirically proved or disproved. And it may simply be my own Christian faith that leads me to reject the plausibility of reincarnation. But I find it very hard to believe that anyone on this earth has ever been here before or will ever be here again. Recent cosmology also supports an analogous interpretation of the life of the universe. Rather than indicating that the universe proceeds (over countless millions of years) in cycles of expansion after a big bang, followed by deceleration and eventual contraction, leading to another big bang, and so on, recent data indicate that the universe is simply expanding continuously and even more rapidly over time, suggesting that there are no cyclic reincarnations of the universe.

10. This is true by virtue of the kind of thing a human being is, even if illness or injury might render a particular individual incapable of expressing one or another of these attributes. Human beings are, as a kind, beings in relationship. Our essence is relational, and this also impacts in an important way on the notion of the personhood of those who are brain damaged. The comatose are still persons because they are damaged individual members of a natural kind of thing that is capable, as a kind, of conscious rationality, desire, and freedom. "Person" is a word we use to designate members of such a kind, not the members of a simple logical class, such that they cease to be members whenever the defining features of the class can no longer be predicated of them. Just as a human being who cannot speak does not cease to be a person (a member of the kind) even though it is characteristic of members of the kind to be able to speak, so a human being who cannot think does not cease to be a person. The terminally ill comatose person has posited the affect, rationality, and freedom of his personhood into the comatose state, and this carries over into death. He does not cease to be a person once he loses the expression of these deeply human capacities. But even those who were *never* conscious belong to the human natural kind and are thus persons because the kind of thing they are (however defective) is characterized by the essential attributes of

persons. Their essence is, in part, defined by their relationship to the rest of us. Although never expressing rationality or freedom as an individual, the never-conscious person (think of an infant born with a fatal brain hemorrhage) still carries with him or her the positing of rationality, affect, and freedom that brought that person into existence and still goes with the individual through the love, attention, and care of parents and those health care professionals who attend to the person's needs. It is the very fact that the person is a member of our kind that makes us able to recognize that he or she is profoundly sick—damaged by virtue of being unable to engage in the attributes that mark members of our kind as persons. We still pick the individual out as a person—a member of our kind—and in virtue of our relationship to that individual as a fellow person we owe him or her our respect and love. Because all of this goes with that person in dying, what I say about human death in general also applies to the death of a premature infant with a fatal brain hemorrhage. See Daniel P. Sulmasy, "Death, Dignity, and the Theory of Value," *Ethical Perspectives* 9 (2003): 103–18, and Daniel P. Sulmasy, "Dignity and the Human as a Natural Kind," in *Health and Human Flourishing*, ed. C. R. Taylor and R. Dell'Oro (Washington, DC: Georgetown University Press, 2006).

11. Rahner, *On the Theology of Death*, 26.

12. Ibid., 51.

13. Ibid., 50.

14. One must be careful not to confuse the transcendent with the transcendental. As Murdoch has put it, "What is transcendent is beyond human experience; what is transcendental is not derived from human experience, but is a condition of it" (Iris Murdoch, *Metaphysics as a Guide to Morals* [New York: Oxford, 1996], 28). This is a subtle, but critical distinction. The transcendental and the transcendent share much in common. Much of what can be said of the transcendent can be said of the transcendental. But the transcendent is metaphysical, whereas the transcendental is epistemological. The transcendent relates to what is beyond the human—the divine, the angelic, the holy other, the supernatural, and the sacred. It is a metaphysical word. It describes a putative ontological possibility. The transcendent is what is beyond ordinary experience, beyond material existence, beyond the possibility of complete comprehension. The transcendental relates to the epistemological preconditions for the possibility of experience, the a priori conditions of knowledge. For instance, the point of Kant's transcendental deduction is that space and time are transcendental—preconditions for the possibility of experience rather than "already out there now" real things.

15. Thomas Aquinas, *Summa Theologiae*, 1-2, q. 50, a. 4, in *Treatise on the Virtues*, trans. J. A. Oesterle (Notre Dame, IN: University of Notre Dame Press, 1966).

16. Sebastian Moore, *The Fire and the Rose Are One* (New York: Seabury, 1980), 26.

17. Aquinas, *Summa Theologiae*, 1-2, q. 60, a. 1.

18. Ibid., q. 63, a. 3, ad. 3.

19. Ibid., q. 62, a. 3.

20. Ibid., q. 62, a. 4.

21. Thomas Merton, *No Man Is an Island* (New York: Harcourt, Brace, Jovanovich, 1955), 17.

22. Monika K. Hellwig, *What Are They Saying about Death and Christian Hope?* (New York: Paulist Press, 1978), 49.

23. Merton, *No Man Is an Island*, 17.

24. Ibid., 18.

25. Ibid., 21.

26. T. S. Elliot, "The *Pensées* of Pascal," in *Selected Essays* (New York: Harcourt, Brace, and Co., 1950), 363.

27. T. S. Eliot, "Ash Wednesday," in *Collected Poems: 1909–1962* (New York: Harcourt, Brace, Jovanovich, 1952), 85.

28. T. S. Eliot, *Four Quartets* (New York: Harcourt, Brace, and World, 1943), 44.

29. Vaclav Havel, *Disturbing the Peace* (New York: Vintage, 1991), 181.

30. Eliot, *Four Quartets*, 28.

31. William F. Lynch, *Images of Hope: Imagination as the Healer of the Hopeless* (Baltimore: Helicon, 1965), 23.

32. Ibid., 24.

33. Ibid., 222 ff.

34. Ibid., 246.

Chapter 12 The Communication of the Dead

1. Jamie Peters, "Attending a Patient's Funeral," *Minnesota Medicine* 87 (January 2004): 32–33.

2. Christine Cassel, "Roundtable Discussion on End of Life Issues," *All Things Considered*, National Public Radio, November 3, 1997.

3. For an example in the self-help category, see Sally D. Miller, *Mourning and Dancing: A Memoir of Grief and Recovery* (Deerfield Beach, FL: Health Communications, 1999). Medical articles documenting the importance of spirituality in coping with grief include P. S. Fry, "The Unique Contribution of Key Existential Factors to the Prediction of Psychological Well-Being of Older Adults following Spousal Loss," *Gerontologist* 41 (2001): 69–81; Kiri Walsh, Michael King, Louise Jones, Adrian Tookman, and Robert Blizard,

"Spiritual Beliefs May Affect Outcome of Bereavement: Prospective Study," *British Medical Journal* 324 (7353) (2002): 1551. However, for a critical review regarding the lack of data documenting the efficacy of interventions to help with grief and loss, see Henk Schut and Margaret S. Stroebe, "Interventions to Enhance Adaptation to Bereavement," *Journal of Palliative Medicine* 8, suppl. no. 1 (2005): S140–47.

4. T. S. Eliot, "Little Gidding," in *Four Quartets* (New York: Harcourt, Brace, and World, 1943), 50–51.

5. Margaret Atwood, "Variations on the Word Sleep," in *Selected Poems 2: Poems Selected and New, 1976–1986* (Boston: Houghton Mifflin, 1987), 77.

6. This is a popular rendering of the Latin *"tu autem eras interior intimo meo,"* perhaps more literally translated by E. B. Pusey as "but Thou wert more inward to me than my most inward part." See St. Augustine. *Confessions of St. Augustine* 3.6.11, trans. E. B. Pusey (New York: Barnes & Noble, 1999). Also available at http://ccat.sas.upenn.edu/jod/augustine/Pusey/book03.

7. Gerard Manley Hopkins, "The Blessed Virgin Compared to the Air We Breathe," in *Gerard Manley Hopkins: Poems and Prose*, ed. W. H. Gardner (Harmondsworth, UK: Penguin, 1953), 55.

8. Cousins, *Bonaventure*, 100.